CUMBRIA COUNTY LIBRARY

LIVING

WITHDRAWN

3 8003 03033 7919

CHALT		
0 2 SEP 2005		
2 5 MAR 2006		
1 3 AUG 2007		
3 0 OCT 2008		
2 5 NOV 2009		
- 3 DEC 2009 *WITHDRAWN*		
2 2 DEC 2009		
1 3 JUL 2010		
- 1 JUL 2011		
1 6 SEP 2014		

616.775   DYSON, S.
LIVING WITH SJOGRENS SYNDROME

Cumbria
COUNTY COUNCIL   **CUM**   D1514108

This book is due to be returne⎯⎯⎯⎯ ⎯ate above. It
may be renewed by personal ap⎯ ⎯⎯⎯ or telephone, if not in
demand.

C.L.18

Overcoming Common Problems Series

Selected titles
A full list of titles is available from Sheldon Press,
36 Causton Street, London SW1P 4ST, and on our website at
www.sheldonpress.co.uk

Overcoming Common Problems Series

Overcoming Common Problems Series

Overcoming Common Problems

Living with Sjögren's Syndrome

Sue Dyson

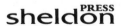

First published in Great Britain in 2005
Sheldon Press
36 Causton Street
London SW1P 4ST

Copyright © Sheldon Press 2005

All rights reserved. No part of this book may be reproduced
or transmitted in any form or by any means, electronic or
mechanical, including photocopying, recording, or by any
information storage and retrieval system, without permission
in writing from the publisher.

The author and publisher have made every effort to ensure that the external website
and email addresses included in this book are correct and up to date at the time of
going to press. The author and publisher are not responsible for the content, quality
or continuing accessibility of the sites.

British Library Cataloguing-in-Publication Data

A catalogue record for this book is available from the British Library

ISBN 0–85969–912–9

1 3 5 7 9 10 8 6 4 2

Typeset by Deltatype Limited, Birkenhead, Merseyside
Printed in Great Britain by Ashford Colour Press

CUMBRIA COUNTY LIBRARY	
H J	15/07/2005
616.775	£7.99

Contents

Acknowledgements

The author and publisher would like to thank Ian Griffiths, consultant rheumatologist at the Freeman Hospital, Newcastle-upon-Tyne, for checking and correcting this book.

Foreword

Chronic diseases are wearing and debilitating. They are even more so when existing medical and surgical treatments can only offer limited benefits. In this situation, sufferers have to search for coping strategies which work for them – and what works today may not work tomorrow, so imagination, tenacity and flexibility are essential. Sjögren's syndrome, named after Dr Henrik Sjögren, a Swedish ophthalmologist who gave the clearest description of the disease in 1933, certainly fits into the above description – and, oddly, may cause additional frustration and irritation for those with the condition in that they often look well but feel awful.

What was recognized 70 years ago was the association of dry eyes and mouth, sometimes in association with arthritis, in an essentially female group of patients. The other key observation was that the affected glands, although showing changes of inflammation, did not have the hallmarks of chronic infection. Some 20 years later the concept of alterations in the body's immune system – so-called auto-immunity – giving rise to these types of disorder started to emerge. It is probably safe to say that if we were starting to define Sjögren's syndrome we 'would not start from here'. Certainly what Henrik Sjögren described in the 1930s can now be categorized into various types and subtypes, and this exercise is not simply an academic nicety; the differing forms have varying clinical and laboratory abnormalities and, more importantly, run differing courses.

The first step is to make the diagnosis and sometimes this can be a somewhat protracted exercise. Although Sjögren's syndrome is not rare, probably affecting about one per cent of the population, it is not a diagnosis that leaps into people's minds. It has not received extensive coverage in the media and, because the symptoms may be vague and non-specific in the early stages, people are often offered alternative explanations such as anxiety or depression.

Certain features of the disease, in particular the dryness of the eyes and mouth, are common to all types, but other features are very much 'tailor made' to the individuals affected. Even within the common strands of dry eyes and mouth, some people find topical lubricants and gels helpful, whereas for others more aggressive therapies are needed. However, it is fair to say that many of the dramatic medical advances which have radically altered the outlook for many of the auto-immune diseases have been singularly disappointing in Sjögren's syndrome and, worse still, often associated with unacceptable side-effects.

In this book, Sue Dyson takes us through the features of the disease and how it expresses itself, illustrating these with her and others' experiences as Sjögren's syndrome sufferers. She also explores thoroughly the various conventional and alternative treatments that are available. Individuals affected by this disease will probably find this 'menu' approach very helpful – some may or may not be relevant to you, and some may not work, but others probably will.

This text provides a balanced introduction to those recently diagnosed and will allow them to frame any questions for the healthcare professional who looks after them. For people with established disease, the range of therapies and strategies described may take them into fruitful avenues not previously explored. Moreover, just reading about how others have coped with chronic disorders may be supportive and enlightening.

This is a book I can thoroughly recommend. It complements other available information literature and explores in great detail many issues which are not covered in often busy and hurried consultations with doctors, dentists and opticians. Remaining positive is critical – chronic illnesses are a bit like gardens: either you are on top of them, or they are on top of you. Rarely is there a comfortable neutral position.

Dr Ian Griffiths

Introduction

Sjögren's syndrome is a somewhat mysterious entity – not much known about and equally hard to pronounce! If you have just been diagnosed with Sjögren's syndrome, the chances are you may never even have heard of it before your doctor gave you a diagnosis. And yet it is estimated that there are around half a million with Sjögren's syndrome in the United Kingdom alone, and 4 million in the USA.

With ever-increasing awareness of auto-immune diseases, however, recognition of Sjögren's syndrome is growing, and some doctors believe that it is more common than initially thought. With its hallmark symptoms of dry eyes and dry mouth, Sjögren's also causes a range of other symptoms that can lead to it being confused with other conditions. For example, aching joints and deep fatigue, two other symptoms, may lead to an initial diagnosis of arthritis – and indeed it is by no means uncommon to be referred to a rheumatologist with arthritis, and then be given a diagnosis of Sjögren's later on. This mirrors the known history of Sjögren's, the discovery of which sprang from a study of patients with arthritis, as described in Chapter 1. Some people too may have Sjögren's in combination with another auto-immune disease, such as lupus. Sjögren's is capable of affecting just about any part of the body. In my own case, for example, it has caused nerve damage to my face (leading to a lopsided smile) and may very well have contributed to my bowel and bladder problems. As my rheumatologist once said: you can blame almost anything on Sjögren's syndrome.

Like many auto-immune disorders, Sjögren's may respond better to a long-term approach that aims at modifying symptoms, rather than an overall cure. The good news is that, for most people, Sjögren's manifests itself in a relatively benign form. Some people may never experience anything more than slightly dry eyes and mouth, which can easily be treated with eye drops, artificial saliva and plenty of fluids. Others may go through days of fatigue but otherwise lead a full life. It is a question of finding out about your individual pattern of Sjögren's, and trying treatments and adapting your lifestyle accordingly.

It does also help to be aware of the potential complications of

Sjögren's. Sometimes this disorder can appear in organs inside the body, and may have a variety of effects, such as digestive disorders (though you should beware of blaming everything on your Sjögren's without having it investigated by a doctor).

On the whole, however, a great deal can be done through self-help, and that is what this book is about. Taking control of your life can help keep you positive and inventive about ways of coping with a long-term condition like Sjögren's. We'll be looking at such areas as your feelings, alternative therapies, relaxation, exercise, nutrition, socializing, pregnancy, family life – all the topics you probably won't get a chance to discuss with your doctor, but which have to be dealt with if you're going to get the best out of life.

This book will also look at the various diagnostic and therapeutic aspects of medical treatment that you can expect to encounter along the way. Perhaps you may just have been diagnosed and may now be wondering exactly how your life will be affected, but that isn't the end of the story. With the help of this book, I hope you will discover that it really is amazing what you can do if you put your mind to it.

(Note: as most people with Sjögren's are women, the person with Sjögren's is usually referred to as 'she' in this book, with some exceptions.)

1
What is Sjögren's syndrome?

Jean
Much of the time I feel fine, if a bit less energetic than I used to be. When my Sjögren's is active, I feel vaguely fluey and really tired and I'll often need to take a few hours' complete rest before my energy comes back. My mouth feels hot and dry and I usually drink lots of iced water. My eyes are very sensitive to light, especially sunlight, and I have to wear sunglasses in all sorts of embarrassing places, such as tube stations, church and concerts! I also have very dry skin and tend to get rashes.

So what is Sjögren's syndrome (pronounced 'Sher-gren' or 'Show-gren')? With its hallmark symptoms of dry eyes, dry mouth, and often fatigue and generalized aching, this condition has only been recognized relatively recently, and certainly isn't a household word yet.

A syndrome is a group of related symptoms or signs that doctors have seen to occur in certain circumstances. This syndrome was described by the Polish doctor Johann Mikulicz-Radecki in 1898, and was at first called Mikulicz syndrome. However, this came to be applied to other conditions which caused dryness and so is no longer used specifically to describe this disease. Sjögren's syndrome (SJS) got its name because this particular set of symptoms was described by Dr Henrik Sjögren, a Swedish ophthalmologist.

In 1933 he noticed that there was a connection in his patients between severe dry eyes, dry mouth and arthritis. Later on, it was recognized that it was also possible for patients to have the dry eyes and mouth without the arthritis. Sjögren described his syndrome in 1933 in his doctoral thesis.

This led to the definition of two kinds of Sjögren's syndrome:

Primary Sjögren's syndrome – Sjögren's syndrome which occurs on its own, with no other associated disease.
Secondary Sjögren's syndrome – Sjögren's syndrome which is associated with another auto-immune disease, such as rheumatoid

arthritis or lupus, or auto-immune liver diseases such as primary biliary cirrhosis.

Sjögren's syndrome and the immune system

Mention of auto-immune disease may raise fears of a weak immune system which may make you prone to disease, but with Sjögren's it would appear that in fact the immune system is over-active.

Almost half a century ago, Sjögren's was defined as a 'chronic auto-immune rheumatic disease characterized by the sicca complex (decreased tears and saliva) and resulting in keratoconjunctivitis sicca (dry eyes) and xerostomia (dry mouth)' (*The New Sjögren's Syndrome Handbook*, 1998; for details see p. 95). Of course, as many Sjögren's patients know only too well, the symptoms can be much more wide-ranging than that, and it is an illness that can attack just about any part of the body. It is very common for patients to suffer from fatigue and aching joints, for example, as well as dry airways and skin; and the disorder can cause problems as diverse as numbness, skin rashes and an under-active thyroid gland.

Inflammation is a common problem, and can affect not only joints but muscles, nerves, kidneys, the thyroid gland and indeed just about any area of the body.

In a Sjögren's patient, instead of the body's immune system attacking invaders, such as germs, it gets mixed up and starts attacking the body's own healthy cells as if they were the invaders. This is called auto (i.e. self) immunity.

This happens in all auto-immune diseases. But in Sjögren's, it is above all the body's moisture-producing glands that the white cells, or lymphocytes, attack and invade. This gradually reduces the glands' ability to produce fluids – tears and saliva – hence the dry eyes and mouth.

During this process, the immune system produces antibodies, exactly as if the body was fighting off a virus. These are called autoantibodies, and through blood tests they can help doctors to diagnose whether or not a patient is suffering from Sjögren's.

Sjögren's is not by any means the only auto-immune disease. There are a whole host of them: some, like lupus and Sjögren's, may affect many organs of the body, while others, like thyroid disease or pernicious anaemia, may single out just one organ. All are related in some way, and sometimes display similar symptoms – which of course complicates the doctor's job of diagnosis. You may find that you are, or have been, tested for some of the following:

- lupus (systemic lupus erythematosus, or SLE);
- scleroderma;
- rheumatoid arthritis;
- polymyositis;
- dermatomyositis;
- thyroid disease;
- auto-immune liver disease.

As we saw earlier, patients with secondary Sjögren's syndrome will also suffer from some other kind of auto-immune disorder, like the ones listed above. Two of the most common include:

Rheumatoid arthritis

Rheumatoid arthritis (RA) is a very common auto-immune disease affecting some one in 100 people, in which the body attacks itself, leading to inflammation and damage to the joints. As the illness is systemic (it affects the whole body) other organs can also be affected, and further symptoms include fatigue and depression.

As with Sjögren's, more women than men are affected. For every man who suffers from this disorder, three women get it, and they also tend to develop it sooner and more severely – it typically manifests first in women in their thirties, and in men in their forties.

Some of the symptoms of rheumatoid arthritis are the same as those that occur in other forms of arthritis and some are quite distinct. As with other auto-immune diseases, experts believe it originates with part of the body's defence system, which attacks the body's own tissue, mistaking it for foreign invaders such as bacteria or viruses. There are more than 100 types of arthritis, not all of which involve inflammation or inflammation alone. Nevertheless, arthritis tends to involve common symptoms including warmth, pain, soreness, tenderness or irritation accompanied by swelling and redness in one or more joints; stiffness in the joint, especially on waking or after inactivity; and difficulty or pain in moving the joint which results in loss of movement and flexibility. Treatment consists of management (rest, pain management, lifestyle changes, and sometimes diet), drugs and in severe cases surgery. Research into RA is ongoing, and areas include genetic inheritance and gene therapy; the role of the hormones (given that so many more women

3

than men contract the disease); the nature of the immune system; and new drugs designed to halt the inflammation process.

Lupus

Lupus is an auto-immune disease in which a person's immune system becomes over-active and attacks the body, causing damage and dysfunction. Lupus is called a multi-system disease because it can reach many different parts of the body, sometimes affecting major body organs.

Some patients with lupus have a very mild condition, which can be treated with simple medications, whereas others can have serious, life-threatening complications. Like Sjögren's, lupus is more common in women – in fact, 90 per cent of sufferers are women – and tends to occur in those between 15 and 40. The reason for this is unknown, as is the cause, though certain factors such as direct sunlight can make the condition worse. As with Sjögren's again, appearances can be deceptive – the typical 'butterfly'-shaped rash on the face gives a false impression of glowing good health while the unfortunate sufferer may be feeling far from healthy.

Symptoms include extreme fatigue, joint pain, muscle aches, anaemia and general malaise, and lupus may mimic other diseases, such as multiple sclerosis and rheumatoid arthritis, making it difficult to diagnose. It is believed to affect more than 30,000 people in the UK and 1.5 million in the USA. Options for lupus sufferers have improved in recent years, with better drug treatments and greater awareness of the condition.

Fibromyalgia – another related condition

Fibromyalgia, sometimes called fibrositis, is a not too well understood group of symptoms involving pain and fatigue, and some estimate that as many as half of all people with Sjögren's also suffer from fibromyalgia. As with Sjögren's and lupus, it can be a frustrating condition in that people often don't look ill but feel awful. Other symptoms include poor or unrefreshing sleep, depression, forgetfulness, poor circulation, headaches including migraine, urgent need to pass water, and irritable bowel type symptoms. Sometimes people with fibromyalgia experience the same kind of debilitating fatigue as those with Sjögren's – an exhaustion that may come on suddenly and necessitate the sufferer putting her feet up for absolute rest.

The pain affects the muscles and ligaments, but not usually the joints, and is often described as a burning kind of pain. Doctors tend to diagnose it by applying pressure to several 'tender points' round the body – in a person with normal health, this may be uncomfortable but not painful; in someone with fibromyalgia, it may cause considerable discomfort or pain.

The cause isn't known, though some research has linked the condition with sleep deprivation. However, it is also thought that a trigger may be needed for fibromyalgia to develop, such as a virus or any incident which poses a trauma to the body – say, childbirth or a car accident. Treatment includes drugs to control the pain and improve sleep, though lifestyle modifications can be very effective in helping people manage their condition: these include rest, diet, exercise, stress management, and warmth or heat to make the body more comfortable.

Symptoms

As we've seen, the two key symptoms of Sjögren's are a dry mouth and dry eyes.

Dry mouth

Julia
On bad days, my mouth sometimes feels as if it's full of cotton wool and I find it more difficult than usual to swallow and taste. Certain foods make my tongue sore, such as tomato ketchup, vinegar, pineapple, orange and apples. My sense of smell has changed, and I have developed a dry cough. I also get occasional mouth infections.

In Sjögren's, the body's immune system gradually attacks and destroys the saliva glands, which are located in the mouth and cheeks and underneath the chin. Most of them are tiny (especially the ones on the inside of your lip), and people don't tend to be aware of them until they stop working properly.

Drinking more helps, but sometimes isn't enough to replace the natural moisture in the mouth because the body is producing diminishing amounts of saliva. Imagine eating ten cream crackers in succession without a drink! This makes eating and swallowing progressively more difficult as the dryness worsens.

Some people may also find that they develop a dry cough, or have difficulty in speaking, and it is quite common to have changes in smell and taste.

Saliva is more than just water. It contains important substances that are designed to help protect the teeth from decay. Consequently, when not enough saliva is present, the result tends to be more dental caries . . . and more tellings-off from the dentist! Indeed, it is often the dentist who spots the first tell-tale signs and recommends the patient to be tested for Sjögren's.

Along with dryness and dental decay comes soreness. A dry mouth easily becomes damaged, cracked and inflamed. Mucous membranes can feel as if they are burning. Infections can get into the gums, and thrush may become a constant problem. In severe cases, the parotid glands on either side of the face (the ones that swell up when you have mumps) can become enlarged, inflamed or infected.

Another complication can be a sore throat and problems with hoarseness in the voice, which can be serious if you have a job like singing or teaching, where you need a good, strong, clear voice. Fortunately, there are ways you can help protect your voice (see Chapter 3).

Dry eyes

Mark

At first I kept running to the mirror to see if I had an eyelash stuck in my left eye, in particular, but there was never anything there. I feel as though there's a bit of sand all the time in my eyes – on a windy day it's as though constant specks of grit are being blown into my eyes. They feel hot and very sensitive.

This is one of the classic signs of Sjögren's – feeling you have a bit of grit in your eye but being unable to see it. As the immune system attacks the glands that produce tears (the lachrymal glands), they produce less and less of the liquid that is vital for lubricating the eyeball. Doctors call this 'aqueous tear deficiency', because the 'water' component of the tears is reduced. Lack of moisture makes the eyes more sensitive to both chemical and physical environmental irritants, producing the gritty sensation. Without tears, the eye's delicate surface is vulnerable to damage every time the eyelid flicks over it, or if a speck of dirt gets in. There may also be an abnormal sensitivity to light, and/or little trails of mucus on the cornea, and the 'white' of the eye may become red. In severe cases, infection and corneal erosions may occur.

Needless to say, a dry eye is also extremely uncomfortable, so most people will seek medical help and advice a long time before any serious damage has been done. I, for example, used to wear soft, disposable contact lenses occasionally, for acting or singing on stage. Gradually I became aware of the fact that they just weren't comfortable any more – they felt gritty, and when I took them out my eyes felt sore. A visit to the optician confirmed that I was not producing enough tears, and I was prescribed eye-drops to replace the moisture.

Is the dryness really due to Sjögren's?

It is important to realize that a number of other conditions can mimic the pattern of the dryness of Sjögren's syndrome, particularly in the early phase. A combination of fatigue, a feeling of dryness and widespread aching may, for example, present as part of depression, fibromyalgia or hypothyroidism.

Other diseases influence the brain centres that control tears and saliva. People with multiple sclerosis and diabetes may have dryness of the eyes and mouth, as these diseases affect the brain processes involved with the control of certain sensory and motor functions.

In addition to problems with the neural activation of the glands, other medical conditions can cause the glands to be dry or to become enlarged. People with fibromyalgia may have fatigue, memory loss, aching muscles and, occasionally, depression. They very frequently have dryness of the eyes and mouth. These symptoms may be very disabling but, unlike in Sjögren's, the gland itself is not damaged. It is important to distinguish them from Sjögren's syndrome itself, which is an auto-immune process that does destroy the gland, since treatment is different.

On top of all this, decreased tear and salivary production occurs as part of the normal ageing process, and a variety of commonly used drugs interfere with the neurogenic stimulus to the tear and salivary glands – the so-called anti-cholinergic drugs. Examples of these would be antidepressants, anti-histamines and some drugs used to treat Parkinson's disease.

Other problems

Mandy

I blamed our old mattress for my discomfort and made my
husband go out and buy an expensive new one – the aches and
pains were just as bad! I sometimes get so tired that I fall asleep
on the sofa watching TV with the kids, and a few times we've
missed their after-school activities, which I feel very guilty about.
I've also got dreadful teeth and have had to have one removed!

Unfortunately, both primary and secondary Sjögren's syndrome can
affect other parts of the body as well, causing problems in the skin,
joints, lungs, kidneys, blood vessels and nervous system – though
usually not all at once! The symptoms are all linked to the immune
system's attack on the body's moisture-producing glands – in other
words, the auto-immune response that causes dry eyes and mouth
can cause inflammation throughout the body.

Even patients with mild primary Sjögren's commonly suffer from
more than just dry eyes and mouth. For example, aching joints and
extreme tiredness are very frequent problems, though not necessarily
as a result of damage caused by the immune system. These
additional problems are known as systemic or extra-glandular
symptoms.

It's important to emphasize that you will probably not have all of
these symptoms. Grouped together as follows, they do make a
fearsome list; however, you are unlikely to have them all and may
indeed only suffer from one or two. Sjögren's can be very
idiosyncratic – part of the reason it's hard to diagnose. Common
other symptoms include:

- Tooth problems. Because saliva helps protect the teeth from
  bacteria, you are more prone to developing cavities if your mouth
  is dry.
- Vision problems. Dry eyes can lead to light sensitivity, blurred
  vision and corneal ulcers.
- Aches and pains. Pain in the muscles and/or joints is common,
  and in many cases is worsened by fibromyalgia, which is thought
  to be a problem for 50–60 per cent of Sjögren's patients and
  which can be extremely debilitating. This kind of pain is also a
  feature of other auto-immune diseases like lupus and rheumatoid
  arthritis and, indeed, some people may have a diagnosis of two of

these, or of all three (whether correctly or not is another matter: diagnosing Sjögren's can be fraught with difficulty as you'll see in Chapter 3, and it has been suggested that some people are over-diagnosed and in fact only have Sjögren's as opposed to two or three auto-immune conditions).

- Extreme fatigue (this can also be a symptom of fibromyalgia). This is not helped by poor sleeping patterns, often due to having to go to the loo several times in the night because of all the extra fluid drunk during the day!
- Dry skin and rashes. About half of those with Sjögren's have dry skin. Some experience only itching, though this can be severe, while others may develop rashes. Others develop cracked, split skin that can easily become infected. Infection is a risk for people with itchy skin, too, particularly if they scratch vigorously.
- Sinusitis and sinus infections. Paradoxically, even when some-one's eyes and mouth are dry, they may suffer postnasal drip. Again, dehydration tends to make this worse.
- Respiratory problems. Some people may suffer upper airway and lung problems such as dry cough, bronchitis or even pneumonia.
- Fever. Some people find that they run a slight temperature – this is often described as 'feeling fluey'.
- Swollen lymph nodes (e.g. in the groin).
- Swollen glands, such as the parotid glands at the side of the face (this may be more common when you are dehydrated).
- Impaired memory and concentration, possibly due to the release of inflammatory substances by the immune system.
- Vaginal dryness. This is common, and some women suffering from it may fail to be diagnosed with Sjögren's. As many cases of Sjögren's start after 40, some women may assume that it is simply part of the menopausal or pre-menopausal process, and so take no action.
- Digestive problems. Difficulty swallowing is often mentioned as a symptom, and this is because the 'dryness' can extend right down into the oesophagus and further into the stomach, pancreas and liver. These internal organs can all suffer from inflammation, resulting in problems like painful swallowing, heartburn and reflux, abdominal pain and swelling, loss of appetite, diarrhoea and irritable bowel syndrome.
- Inflammatory problems with internal organs such as heart, liver and, most commonly, the kidneys.

• Nerve problems. Inflammation can sometimes attack the nerves in the arms, legs or extremities, causing problems such as pain, numbness and tingling in the fingers (which may be due to carpal tunnel syndrome); in the legs or arms (due to a peripheral neuropathy); or in the face or throat (cranial neuropathy).

Sjögren's syndrome and lymphoma?

Many people with Sjögren's worry about developing cancer of the lymph nodes, or lymphoma. The early studies into Sjögren's syndrome in the 1960s found that lymphoma occurred 44 times more commonly than in age- and sex-matched people without the syndrome. However, in those days some of the treatments for Sjögren's, for example X-ray irradiation for swollen parotid glands, may have further enhanced the risk of lymphoma. Subsequent studies, however, while confirming the increased risk of lymphoma, have shed further light on this worrying aspect. Only a subset of patients with Sjögren's are at increased risk, and these are the patients with particular abnormal antibodies, known as the Ro and La antibodies (see p. 16). Patients with secondary Sjögren's, or those with only the dry eyes or mouth and without the abnormal antibodies, do not have an increase in lymphoma. Moreover, in those people who are unlucky enough to develop lymphoma, it is often at the very mild end of the lymphoma spectrum, sometimes known as a maltoma. In fact, these lymphomas often follow such a mild course that the specialists, usually haematologists or oncologists, may well decide not to treat them but merely keep them under observation. Overall, in a ten-year period lymphoma may develop in about 5 per cent of those who have both the syndrome and the immunological abnormalities.

The most common symptom of lymphoma is a painless swelling of the lymph nodes in the neck, underarm or groin. The salivary glands may also be swollen, usually in an asymmetrical fashion. Other symptoms may include fever, night sweats, constant fatigue, unexplained weight loss, itchy skin and red patches on the skin. However, these can be due to a host of other factors apart from lymphoma, so do consult your doctor for advice and diagnosis. Ultimately the diagnosis rests on obtaining a biopsy from the suspect site. This also allows the lymphoma (if that is what is found) to be classified as within the mild or more aggressive end of the spectrum, and the appropriate treatment planned.

Who gets Sjögren's syndrome?

Sjögren's can affect anybody, male or female, young or old, and from any ethnic background. However, if there is such a thing as a 'typical' Sjögren's patient, she is probably middle-aged and female. It is common for the disease to develop (or be diagnosed) around the age of 40 or over, and it is estimated that only around one in ten patients are male. It has been estimated that around one in every 500 people has Sjögren's.

Nobody is sure why Sjögren's attacks mainly women, but it is possible that female hormones such as oestrogen are involved in making women more liable to develop the disease.

There is some evidence that a predisposition to Sjögren's may run in families. Other auto-immune diseases – particularly lupus and thyroid problems – are also more common among the relatives of people with Sjögren's.

Scientists are pretty sure that there is a genetic component to Sjögren's syndrome. Genes known as HLA (human leukocyte antigen) genes are involved in controlling the immune response and are inherited, just like the genes for eye colour or curly hair. One gene, called HLA-DR3, is frequently found in white people with primary Sjögren's, and other genes are associated with the disorder in different ethnic groups. However, there are likely to be multiple genes involved, and at this stage it is too early to state definitely which particular genes these are.

So, while it may be possible to inherit a genetic predisposition to Sjögren's syndrome, merely having the right combination of genes (and, remember, we don't yet know what they are) does not guarantee you will develop full-blown Sjögren's. Many relatives will test positive for the antibodies present in Sjögren's, but will never develop any of the symptoms.

It is thought that a genetic predisposition alone is not enough to produce the disease, and that there may also have to be a trigger. As yet, scientists are not quite sure what that trigger is, but there is evidence to suggest that – in some cases at least – it may be a viral

11

infection. In my own case, for example, I developed a throat infection shortly before the first symptoms of Sjögren's syndrome manifested themselves. Another sufferer I know developed symptoms after a severe bout of flu. Some researchers have suggested that the Epstein-Barr virus (the cause of glandular fever) may be the culprit, but there is as yet no proof of this. Again, no consistent pattern emerges around the globe. For example, in Japan an illness very similar to Sjögren's is associated with a virus that can cause a rare form of leukaemia – the HTLV1 virus – but this association is not found anywhere else. In countries bordering the Mediterranean, a link between the hepatitis C virus and Sjögren's has been observed, but this hasn't been found in other parts of the world.

Preventing Sjögren's

While symptoms are often treatable, there is no way of preventing Sjögren's syndrome. But early diagnosis and intervention can prevent complications. As already stated in the Introduction, self-help measures can go a long way towards making you more comfortable, while regular medical check-ups can help monitor any changes in symptoms.

2
Diagnosing Sjögren's syndrome

It can take a long time to get a diagnosis of Sjögren's syndrome, because, as described in the previous chapter, people can display a wide variety of symptoms, and this may make it difficult for doctors to arrive at a conclusive diagnosis. One of the great frustrations of Sjögren's is that people look well but feel awful. It is not uncommon to take a roundabout route to eventual diagnosis. My own doctor had just prescribed eye-drops for my dry eyes when my dentist noticed the excessive dryness in my mouth, put two and two together and sent me off for further tests which eventually resulted in a diagnosis of Sjögren's.

Julia had suffered for several months with various complaints including aching joints, sore eyes and sweating attacks. As described in Chapter 1, like many other people she was referred to the rheumatology department of her local hospital, receiving a subsequent diagnosis of Sjögren's only months later.

Another potential complication is that the symptoms that characterize Sjögren's syndrome can also indicate several other illnesses. Even those with Sjögren's may not realize that there is a connection between their gritty eyes and their parched mouths, their itching skin and their joint problems. Some GPs may not be very well informed about the condition and may also fail to spot the pattern, instead trying to treat the individual symptoms as separate problems or beginning investigations into other diseases.

A sympathetic GP may refer a patient to a specialist for one of the problems – perhaps an ophthalmologist for the dry eyes, or an ENT consultant for problems with a dry mouth and hoarseness of voice. Or perhaps you yourself may consult your dentist about problems such as inflamed gums, a dry tongue or tooth decay.

Your doctor will probably ask you about any other symptoms you may have. An informed GP may look for other signs of Sjögren's, such as red itchy eyes, swollen salivary glands, a dry cracked tongue, and enlarged salivary glands in your neck. You'll also want to discuss what medications you are taking – both prescription and over-the-counter – as many medications can exacerbate oral dryness, notably:

- tricyclic antidepressants;
- monoamine oxidase inhibitors;
- muscle-relaxing agents;
- blood pressure medications;
- heart medication;
- anti-seizure drugs.

Once these factors have been eliminated, your doctor may arrange a series of diagnostic tests, including some of the following.

The Schirmer test

The Schirmer test is a simple test for dry eyes. A strip of sterile filter paper (a bit like blotting paper) is inserted between the eyeball and the lower eyelid and left there for five minutes. When it is removed, the doctor measures how much of the strip is wet (a normal reading is usually in excess of 8 mm per five minutes). This indicates whether the lachrymal glands are producing enough tears or not.

Tests using dyes

These tests are carried out by eye specialists (ophthalmologists) using slit lamp imaging to detect changes. The doctor can assess whether the eye has been damaged by the diminished output of tears by inserting a drop of dye (rose bengal or fluorescein). The dye clings briefly to any dry/damaged areas, making it possible to identify them more easily.

Mouth examination

The doctor will look into the mouth for signs of dryness and will check to see if any of the main salivary glands (parotid, submandibular, sublingual) are swollen. Tell-tale signs of dryness include:

- dry, sticky mouth;
- smooth-looking tongue;
- redness;
- dental decay;
- little, or very thick, saliva;

- dry, cracked lips;
- sores at the corners of the mouth.

A simple screening test used in the clinic is to collect the saliva production over a defined period by getting the person to spit all saliva formed into a measuring container. Normally this should be more than 1.5 ml in 15 minutes. The doctor may also try to stimulate saliva production by massaging the glands or administering a sour substance. Cloudy saliva can indicate the presence of infection.

Saliva manufactured by the parotid glands (the ones that make you look like a hamster when you have mumps) enters the mouth via two tiny openings inside the mouth, next to the upper molars on either side. These openings are called Stenson's ducts. If the doctor wishes to check the flow of saliva, a suction-cup can be placed over the opening and the amount of saliva measured.

It is also possible to image the salivary glands using ultrasound, MRI or radioactive isotopes, but these tests are not commonly used in everyday practice.

Lip biopsy

To be extra sure that a patient has Sjögren's syndrome, a lip biopsy may be carried out. Often this is done on an outpatient basis in the oral surgery department of the local hospital. It is a short procedure, usually done under local anaesthetic with the patient sitting up in a dentist's chair, during which one of the tiny minor salivary glands is removed from inside the lower lip.

The gland is then examined in the pathology department, to see if it is inflamed and whether it has been invaded by lymphocytes (white cells), both indications that Sjögren's syndrome may be present.

Blood tests

As discussed earlier, Sjögren's patients manufacture specific antibodies in their blood and blood tests are frequently used to diagnose the condition. These tests will also help doctors to eliminate other possibilities, such as rheumatoid arthritis or lupus. Doctors will be testing for:

15

Autoantibodies

Antinuclear antibodies

These antibodies are classically found in all patients with lupus but also occur commonly in patients with Sjögren's, being present in up to 70 per cent in some groups of patients. The antinuclear antibodies represent a family of antibodies, and nowadays we are able to test for the presence or absence of individual members, two of which – Ro and La – are particularly important in Sjögren's.

Ro and La

Also known as SS-A and SS-B, these are antinuclear antibodies that are frequently found in the blood of Sjögren's sufferers. Ro antibodies are found in 60–70 per cent of patients, while La antibodies are found in around 40 per cent, particularly those with primary Sjögren's.

Ro antibodies can also be present in people with other auto-immune disorders, so on their own they do not necessarily confirm the presence of Sjögren's syndrome. Also, it is possible to have Sjögren's without having these antibodies.

Other antinuclear antibodies are found in the blood of people with lupus but can also be present in Sjögren's patients – so on their own they do not mean that a patient is suffering from lupus.

Rheumatoid factor

This is the name given to a group of antibodies that are found not only in the blood of people with rheumatoid arthritis, but sometimes in people who have other auto-immune diseases, including Sjögren's syndrome. On its own it does not mean that an individual has rheumatoid arthritis.

Often it is the finding of both an antinuclear antibody and rheumatoid factor on a screening test that alerts a doctor to the possibility of Sjögren's.

Markers of inflammation

The commonest screening test measures the erythrocyte sedimentation rate (ESR). A normal result is less than 20 mm, increasing if there is inflammation for any reason, so this test is fairly non-specific but sensitive. If an individual's ESR is high, for example over 50, it may indicate that that person has Sjögren's syndrome or a connective tissue disease. Interestingly, another frequently measured marker of inflammation, the C reactive protein, is not raised in Sjögren's, so this discrepancy again may suggest Sjögren's.

Immunoglobulins

These are normal antibodies (proteins) that help protect the body from disease. If a person has Sjögren's, their levels are usually high. Levels can vary according to how active a patient's Sjögren's is at any given time, so once you have been diagnosed your doctor may wish to carry out this test at regular intervals.

Other tests

In addition to all these blood tests, it is possible that your doctor may wish you to have a chest X-ray, as in rare cases Sjögren's can cause inflammation of the lungs. You may also have a urine test, to see how well your kidneys are functioning. Once you are on medication, you will probably have regular blood tests to track the progress of your illness, and in some cases to check that the medicines you are taking are not harming your liver, kidneys, etc.

Today, there is a broad international consensus on the diagnosis of Sjögren's syndrome. There is no single diagnostic test and the diagnosis depends upon fulfilling five out of six sets of criteria. Two relate to symptoms of dry eyes or mouth, and two more are to do with objective evidence of impaired tear or salivary secretion. The remaining two are the specific Ro or La antibodies in the blood and an abnormal lip biopsy.

What happens next?

A diagnosis can be reassuring, ending a period of uncertainty and suspense. Now that you have a name to put to your condition, you can start to get to grips with it. This means getting to know your illness and the best ways of managing it, which may be a matter of trial and error, along with advice and help from your doctor. The next chapter looks at some of the medical treatments available to combat Sjögren's syndrome.

3

Treating Sjögren's syndrome
– simple measures

The simplest treatments are often the most effective, and are certainly the ones least likely to cause unwanted side-effects. It is likely that your GP or specialist will begin by trying you on some of these simple approaches, in the hope that the more complex (and potentially more problematic) drug treatments won't become necessary. (We look at these in the next chapter.)

Simple solutions to a dry mouth

Xerostomia – the chronic dry mouth characteristic of Sjögren's patients – can be distressing, and in severe cases it can make swallowing unduly difficult.

Solutions need to keep the mouth and throat reasonably moist, without harmful side-effects such as dental decay. Sugary sweets and drinks may stimulate the flow of saliva, for instance, but they're hardly a good idea when the downside is rampant caries and obesity!

Luckily, a variety of sugar-free sweets are now available, and used in moderation these can be very valuable in stimulating failing saliva glands to increase production. You will probably find that sour substances, like lemon and vinegar, also tend to make your mouth water, but be careful – lemon too can cause tooth erosion.

Julia favoured small sips of cider vinegar diluted with water, as her grandmother had often recommended it as a home remedy for fatigue, arthritis and every ailment under the sun!

Sugarless chewing gum is another good standby and can be chewed throughout the day. And, of course, there is that good old favourite, plain drinking water – if you want to avoid frequent trips to the lavatory, try rinsing your mouth with the water rather than swallowing it.

The standard medical treatment for a dry mouth is artificial saliva. This comes in tubes or spray bottles, either as a colourless, slightly sticky gel or as a rather slimy liquid. Some people say that the gel

18

lasts a little longer than the liquid, as it adheres better to the inside of the mouth. Like real saliva, the liquid is liable to be swallowed, but this doesn't really matter as artificial saliva can be used as many times as needed. Artificial saliva can be prescribed or bought over the counter at your local pharmacy. Products containing fluoride are best.

More tips

- Avoid eating foods that can dry or irritate your mouth, such as nuts, chocolate, strong cheeses and shellfish.
- You can soothe dry, cracked lips by using oil- or petroleum-based lip balm or lipstick.
- If your mouth hurts, the doctor may give you medicine in a mouth rinse, ointment or gel to apply to the sore areas to control pain and inflammation.
- Drink fluids throughout the day, but instead of drinking large amounts of water, which can cause excessive urination, try drinking small sips of water and rinsing your mouth frequently.
- Try sucking on chips of ice or frozen grapes. Some people have also found grape juice helpful, especially when held in the mouth for a few moments before being swallowed.
- A diet rich in raw fruits and vegetables will stimulate the parasympathetic nervous system and reduces acidity in the mouth and stomach, which in turn can help stimulate saliva.
- Tea and coffee are diuretic and add to drying, so are best avoided. Try weak versions, or drink herbal teas instead.
- Try to breathe through the nose rather than open-mouth breathing. A soft cervical collar, used while sleeping, may prevent open-mouth breathing by supporting the jaw. Sleep in a cool bedroom and avoid air conditioning if possible.

Check your mouth

Only a minority of people with a painful or burning mouth will actually develop thrush, a candida infection characterized by white patches inside the mouth or as red, burning areas in the mouth. However, if you do feel you could have symptoms of a mouth infection, or if your usual symptoms deteriorate and you have a painful mouth and burning tongue, do have them looked at by your doctor or dentist.

It is a good idea to check your mouth regularly, so that you know what is normal for you and are more likely to notice if you do develop unusual redness, other colouration, mouth pain or bleeding. If you do develop thrush, you may find that bathing the mouth with live yoghurt is soothing; otherwise, your doctor can prescribe antifungal drugs. These can be taken in tablet form and may take a couple of weeks to work. Various viruses and bacteria can also cause infections and these can be treated with antiviral or antibiotic medicines.

Oral hygiene

Julia

I have lost one tooth and am taking great care of the rest! I have got to know my dentist and hygienist quite well – they understand my Sjögren's and are very helpful with advice on cleaning, check-ups and so on. So far I've avoided losing any more teeth.

Good oral hygiene is vital in Sjögren's. Saliva contains substances that get rid of the mouth bacteria that cause cavities and infections, and of course, if this decreases problems can develop. In Sjögren's, tooth decay is common, and some people may also suffer mouth infections. For many, it can be helpful to cultivate a good relationship with their dentist and oral hygienist, who can build up a knowledge of their mouths and condition.

- Visit your dentist regularly to have your teeth examined and cleaned.
- Rinse your mouth with water several times a day. Don't use a mouthwash that contains alcohol because alcohol is drying.
- Brush your teeth immediately before and after eating, as well as before bedtime. Brushing before meals helps to eliminate oral bacteria that might cling to food particles and encourage decay. Electric toothbrushes may be helpful.
- Avoid sticky, sugary foods. Eating fewer sweet treats results in less acid in the mouth and reduces the risk of tooth decay. Three teaspoons of sugar eaten only once daily is less detrimental to tooth enamel than one teaspoon of sugar consumed at three different times. Every time sugar is introduced into the diet, bacteria produce acid for 20 minutes.
- Avoid acidic foods, including citrus fruits, which can damage tooth enamel.

- If drinking soft drinks, choose sugar-free varieties and use a straw to protect the teeth from acidity.
- You might find it soothing to apply the contents of a vitamin E capsule to your mouth, especially at night.
- A mouthwash prepared from a quarter of a teaspoon of baking soda dissolved in a quarter of a cup of warm water can reduce oral acidity and produce a fresh taste in the mouth.
- Don't use toothpaste designed for stained teeth because it might be too harsh on your tooth enamel. Use fluoride toothpaste to gently brush your teeth, gums and tongue.
- Floss your teeth every day. Small brushes are also very effective for cleaning between the teeth.
- Avoid sugar. That means choosing sugar-free gum, candy and soda. If you do eat or drink sugary foods, brush your teeth immediately afterwards.
- Ask your dentist whether you need to take fluoride supplements, use a fluoride gel at night, or have a protective varnish put on your teeth to protect the enamel.

Simple solutions to dry eyes

Your doctor will probably recommend a simple treatment in the form of artificial tears. Like artificial saliva, this is a product designed to mimic the natural substance as closely as possible; but of course it isn't as good, because it tends to drain away and then has to be replaced manually. Nevertheless, if you have dry, gritty eyes, artificial tears are an absolute godsend: they can remove the discomfort almost instantly.

There are two different forms: liquid drops, which come in a squeezy bottle, and gel tears, which come in a small tube. You simply pull the lower eyelid slightly forward and squeeze a few drops on to the surface of the eye. Blinking will spread the fluid over the eyeball.

The choice of drops or gel is a matter of personal preference, and it may be worth experimenting if one type does not help. Sometimes people become sensitized to the preservative in normal artificial tears, and this is a particular problem in people who have had their naso-lachrymal ducts blocked. They start to notice that the eyes sting when the drops are used, and then preservative-free drops are needed. I personally rather like the gel tears, as I find they last a good long time, but on the down side they are quite thick and have a tendency to blur the vision for a short while after insertion. For this reason they may work best if you use them at night, so there is less burning, dryness and itching when you wake up in the morning. Artificial tears can be prescribed or bought over the counter at a pharmacy.

Other eye-protection tips

- Protect your eyes from the wind. Don't direct hairdryers towards your eyes, and let your hair dry naturally when possible so you can avoid their use. Avoid drafts from air conditioners, heaters and radiators when possible.
- Use goggles when swimming.
- Avoid smoky or dusty atmospheres.
- Keep makeup away from your eyes. Apply mascara only to the tips of your lashes so it doesn't get in your eyes. If you use eyeliner or eye shadow, put it only on the skin above your lashes, not on the sensitive skin under your lashes, close to your eyes.
- Use wraparound sunglasses to help protect your eyes from the sun, wind and dust.
- Blink several times a minute while reading or working on the computer.
- Avoid rubbing your eyes, however strong the temptation is to do so.
- Put a humidifier in the rooms where you spend the most time, including the bedroom, or install a humidifier in your heating and air conditioning unit.
- Ask your doctor whether any of your medications contribute to dryness and, if so, how to reduce that effect.
- Consider soft contact lenses rather than the traditional hard ones, though many patients with Sjögren's are unable to wear contact lenses at all.

Treating dry eye with petroleum jelly

The eye's tear film has three layers:

- a mucin layer next to the eyeball;
- a tear (aqueous) on top of the mucin layer;
- floating on these two layers, a lipid (fatty, oily) layer, which prevents the tear layer evaporating.

In Sjögren's syndrome, dry eyes result from problems in both the tear and the lipid layer. Not only do Sjögren's patients make insufficient tears, their tears also evaporate faster than they should because of an inadequate lipid layer, so compounding the problem. This problem has been tackled in an interesting way with the help of that humble substance, petroleum jelly. According to research by Dr Donald MacKeen of the Sjögren's Syndrome Foundation, Bethesda, USA, petroleum jelly placed next to the eye helps reduce dryness and the blink rates of patients. This so-called 'supracutaneous effect' is due to the fact that the jelly gradually spreads or 'migrates' into the surrounding eyeskin, supposedly reducing soreness and dryness.

A controlled study reported in the *British Journal of Ophthalmology* tested this theory. Researchers Dr Kazuo Tsubota and colleagues of the Tokyo Dental College, Chiba, Japan, found that participants reported significant improvement in dry eye symptoms when calcium carbonate in a petroleum ointment was applied to the lower eyelids.

From anecdotal reports, it would also appear that petroleum jelly causes less burning and less tearing of the skin around the eye, with less need for artificial tears, goggles or protective glasses – though you may look a little shiny around the eye! It is recommended that, for best results, the product you try is 100 per cent pure petroleum.

If you try this, here are some tips:

- Start off with a small blob of jelly and don't apply too near the eye – a little outside the lashline.
- Use a cotton bud or clean finger to apply.
- Some people recommend that you treat both upper and lower lids, applying an extra amount at bedtime and during the night.
- Expect some blurring. It may be best to experiment with this at bedtime.

Simple solutions to aches and pains

Joint pain can be a fact of life for people with Sjögren's. The good news is that over-the-counter painkillers can be used to very good effect in many cases. The main non-prescription analgesics are: paracetamol, combinations of paracetamol and codeine, and ibuprofen.

Ibuprofen is an anti-inflammatory drug and particularly good for arthritic-type pain, although paracetamol is generally kinder on the stomach. If you suffer from stomach trouble (ulcers, gastritis, bleeding, etc.), you should check with your doctor that it is all right for you to take these types of drug. You can also buy pain-relieving creams and gels based on ibuprofen and other anti-inflammatory drugs, for example:

- ibuprofen gel;
- Nurofen gel;
- Voltarol emulgel.

These are effective for treating localized pain – for example, a sore shoulder or knee. It is said that the concentration of the drug that reaches the individual trouble-spot is much greater if gel is rubbed on the skin than if a painkiller is taken orally.

Again, these products are available over the counter, but your doctor may also prescribe them for you. It is worth establishing whether the cost of the prescription would be higher than the cost of buying the drug over the counter.

Simple solutions to skin problems

To treat dry skin, apply heavy moisturizing creams and ointments three or four times a day to trap moisture in the skin. Lotions, which are lighter than creams and ointments, aren't recommended because they evaporate quickly and can actually contribute to dry skin.

Take a quick shower (less than five minutes), use a moisturizing soap, pat your skin almost dry, and then cover it with a cream or ointment at once. If you prefer a bath, put some emollient oil in and then allow a few minutes' soaking to give your skin time to absorb moisture. Avoid prolonged hot showers or baths.

Other tips

- For particularly dry patches of skin, talk to your health care professional about using emollients containing salicylic acid, lactate or urea. For itching, your doctor might recommend that you use a skin cream or ointment containing steroids.
- Place a humidifier (and an air purifier, if you feel it helps) in your

home and at work to increase your comfort, keeping humidity between 30 and 50 per cent. You may want to use a humidifier year-round. Some experts advise using a cool-mist, ultrasonic humidifier; be sure to clean it daily.

- Use a nasal rinse or spray made of water and salt to alleviate a dry nose and nasal congestion.
- If you have nasal and airway dryness, consider using a soft cervical collar while you sleep to discourage your mouth from opening, thus preventing the dryness that mouth breathing causes.
- Use moisturizing skin creams or ointments throughout the day.
- Use only moisturizing soaps while bathing. Avoid antibacterial soaps or abrasive cleansers.
- After bathing, don't dry your skin completely. Leave a film of moisture and then moisturize with a cream or ointment. Emollients with urea, lactate or salicylic aid help in sloughing off dead skin and allowing a healthier, softer skin to emerge.
- Your skin may be extra-sensitive to the sun, especially if you also have lupus, and may burn from even a little exposure. Cover your skin when outside, and use a sunscreen with a good SPF (sun protection factor), 15 or stronger. Also wear protective clothing such as long-sleeved t-shirts and headwear, and try to avoid being in the sun for long periods of time.
- Coat your lips with petroleum-based lubricants to prevent drying. (Many lipsticks can provide this protection.)
- Consider installing a water conditioner if you live in a hard-water area.
- Talk to your health care professional about discontinuing your use of decongestants and anti-histamines because they dry your mouth and nasal areas.
- If you suffer from nosebleeds or sinus problems, try gently hosing your nose with a saline mix (a mix of water and salt which you can prepare yourself at home).

Simple solutions for other problem areas

Vaginal dryness

Vaginal dryness may be one of the more embarrassing effects of Sjögren's syndrome. Indeed, some women may fail to be diagnosed because they assume this is a symptom of menopause that they have to 'put up with'. A vaginal moisturizing product or lubricant may help relieve discomfort. Sustained use of lubricants can, however, disrupt the normal mucosa of the vagina, making lubricants inappropriate for long-term application. Instead, you may find vitamin E pessaries helpful. During the first month of use, insert the pessary into the vagina once a day; after several months, one suppository one to three times a week may be enough.

Swollen glands

A swollen face and jaw, and sometimes toothache and headache, are common symptoms of an inflamed gland. If you suffer from these, try massaging the swollen gland and applying heat. Sucking on hard sugarless sweets may also help.

Cold extremities

Some people with Sjögren's suffer cold hands and feet due to impaired circulation. In particular, some may suffer from Raynaud's syndrome, when the fingers and toes go numb and white, caused by spasm of the arteries which take blood to these areas. This often takes place in the cold. Keep gloves handy for cold jobs like removing items from the fridge and freezer, or going outside into the garden. Thermal mitts and socks may help. A warm hat is also helpful to help retain heat in the body.

Protecting your voice

People with Sjögren's can develop hoarseness if their vocal cords become inflamed as part of the disease or become irritated from throat dryness or coughing. To prevent further strain on your vocal cords, try not to clear your throat before speaking. Instead, take a sip of water, chew gum or suck on candy. Or else make an 'h' sound, hum or laugh to gently bring the vocal cords together so you can get sound out. Clearing your throat does the same thing, but it's hard on the vocal cords and you want to avoid irritating them further.

4

Treatment – medication

Unfortunately, as mentioned before, there isn't as yet any cure for Sjögren's. What doctors can do is to treat the various symptoms, individually or collectively. The good news is that in most patients – particularly those with primary Sjögren's – treatment works well, without too many side-effects.

Incidentally, you'll note that I say 'specialist' rather than 'rheumatologist', because although most Sjögren's patients are looked after by a rheumatologist, all kinds of people from different specialisms may be involved in your treatment. For example:

- dentist;
- oral surgeon;
- ENT specialist;
- ophthalmologist (eye specialist);
- orthoptist (professional who deals with abnormal eye movements);
- pain relief specialist.

Although it can be useful to have the benefit of different people's skills and perspectives, I sometimes think that, with so many different specialists involved, things can get unnecessarily complicated and wires can become crossed. In my own case, for example, I have seen all of the above at one time or another; but when I have suddenly become acutely ill, nobody has been quite sure which department I come under or who ought to decide whether I'm admitted to hospital – and if so, to which ward!

It would be ideal if all the medical professionals involved in your care could meet and discuss the different symptoms and problems together. Or, even better, if there could be dedicated Sjögren's clinics all over the country, where professionals from different disciplines could work together closely and exchange information on patients. Until that day, the best you can do is to inform yourself about your condition so that you can approach the right professional, for the right treatment, at the right time.

27

More complex medication

The products we have been looking at are all an important part of the anti-Sjögren's armoury. There are few Sjögren's patients who haven't used at least some of them on a regular basis. But when things are a little worse than the odd bit of grittiness in the eye, the slightly dry mouth or the occasional twinge in a joint, doctors have access to much more powerful forms of treatment. The negative side of these drugs is that they are liable to produce more undesirable side-effects than simpler, non-prescription remedies.

Medication for dry mouth

It is worth mentioning again, I think, that there are some drugs that can make a dry mouth worse. Your doctor should run through everything you are taking, to ensure that you are not contributing to your own condition.

Examples of drugs that may make oral dryness worse are antidepressants, tricyclic analgesics (such as amitriptyline), anti-histamines and beta blockers.

It is possible to prescribe certain drugs, for example pilocarpine, that stimulate increased salivary flow. Pilocarpine has been shown to be effective in clinical trials with patients who still have some function in their salivary glands. It doesn't suit everybody, however. Some people can develop side-effects such as sweating, urinary frequency, dizziness and flushing, but these can often be overcome by starting on a small dose and increasing the dose gently over a period of weeks, and if need be stopping on a less than maximal dose. How useful it is in individual people is best found out by trying it and seeing whether or not it suits them personally.

Other oral problems

As we've seen, fungal infections and dental caries are common problems when the mouth is dry. Another occupational hazard for Sjögren's people is the possibility of infections or blockages in the major saliva glands.

I once developed a very strange bulge under my tongue. When I lifted my tongue, it looked as if I had a pink glassy bauble on the floor of my mouth. It turned out that this was the result of a blocked sublingual gland, which had to be removed by surgery. It is a good idea to remove a blocked gland of this type because there is always a slight chance of malignancy. But in most cases – like mine – it is a simple calcium deposit, caused by a thickening of the saliva. When the saliva glands become infected – particularly the parotid glands, at the sides of the face and neck – they tend to become sore and swell up, giving a mumps-like appearance. The saliva may also become thick and infected. If this happens, a course of antibiotics will probably put things right quite quickly. Only in rare cases do glands have to be removed.

Anti-inflammatory medication

Inflammation in the body increases when Sjögren's becomes more active, and there are drugs that can help to combat this. Among the most commonly used are nonsteroidal anti-inflammatory drugs, known as NSAIDs.

NSAIDs don't just reduce inflammation (as in arthritis); they also reduce pain. In many ways they are similar to aspirin and ibuprofen, and so their side-effects are similar too: in particular there is a risk of stomach irritation and/or bleeding. In severe cases, sensitive patients could even develop a peptic ulcer. Some people cannot tolerate NSAIDs but most can, especially with careful use and the help of drugs that protect the stomach. These include lansoprazole (Zoton). Over-the-counter remedies such as Gaviscon can also help.

Modern anti-inflammatories such as Celebrex are kinder to the stomach than the older drugs; and another way to reduce the chance of problems is to administer the drug in suppository form. I know many British people turn green at the very thought of a suppository, but I use Voltarol suppositories, and believe me, they're a godsend. They get the drug into the bloodstream more quickly than tablets, and do not have such an irritant effect on the stomach.

Immuno-suppressant and anti-rheumatic medication

As we've seen, Sjögren's is very much a disorder of the immune system – an over-active immune system, in fact. So one of the ways in which doctors treat it is to try to suppress that over-activity.

The first line of immuno-suppressant medication is steroids. The most commonly prescribed steroid is prednisolone, which is generally given in tablet form but can be administered by drip if you are in hospital and the dose is a large one. Like NSAIDs, steroids can have an irritant effect on the stomach, so they are often prescribed in the form of enteric-coated tablets. This means that they have a coating that does not dissolve until the tablet is safely out of the stomach and into the intestine.

Steroids are of help to some Sjögren's people. But they are strong drugs, with undesirable side-effects, and if possible it is better to use them just for flare-ups rather than continuously. This is because long-term use can lead to such diverse problems as osteoporosis, peptic ulcer, diabetes, fragile skin, poor wound healing and eye troubles.

There is also the problem that everyone immediately thinks of when steroids are mentioned: weight gain. Putting on huge amounts of weight isn't inevitable, but the fact that steroids increase the appetite doesn't exactly help! They also promote water retention, and tend to produce a plump, round-faced appearance which can be embarrassing. I know I've struggled with my weight since I started on steroids, and would dearly love not to have to take them. But unfortunately, every time the dose is reduced I have another flare-up. So for the time being at least, I'm just grateful that there's something I can take to ease the pain.

Eating sensibly is very important – not just because of the risk of weight gain, but to guard against bone problems. Your doctor can advise you on a good, bone-strengthening diet with lots of calcium and green vegetables, but you may also wish to take a mineral supplement specifically designed to promote bone health. Today, most doctors will also prescribe some form of therapy to try and avoid osteoporosis if you are likely to be taking steroids for more than a few weeks – the commonly used agents are the bisphospho-nate drugs or calcium and vitamin D compounds. Women who are past the menopause, or who – like me – have had their ovaries removed, may be wise to take some form of treatment to protect their bones, but this is an issue you will need to discuss with your doctor, to determine whether it is the right course of action for you.

Anti-rheumatic medication generally does not help Sjögren's, with the exception of hydroxychloroquine which has some modest benefit in improving fatigue and joint pain, according to laboratory tests. It is very slow acting and people may need to take it for six months before seeing any benefit.

The more powerful immuno-suppressant drugs, like azathioprine, cyclosporin and methotrexate, do not help Sjögren's.

Drugs designed to control chronic pain

Of course, specific anti-inflammatory or immuno-suppressant medication cannot always solve the problem, and some people will be left with some degree of chronic pain. Others may have periodic flare-ups when things seem to get out of control and the pain starts taking over.

This is when your local pain clinic comes into its own. We'll look into this in more detail in Chapter 6, when we discuss self-help and pain management programmes, but as we're talking about medication this seems a good point to mention some of the drugs that can be used to treat chronic pain.

Unlike acute pain, chronic (long-lasting) pain can't easily be wiped out with a couple of painkillers. The messages between the brain and the nerves can become garbled, and other medication may work more efficiently in sorting this out.

Some of the drugs commonly used in pain clinics are:

- gabapentin: originally an anti-epilepsy drug, but found to be an effective pain suppressant;
- carbamazepine;
- amitriptyline: an old-style tricyclic antidepressant, rarely used these days for the treatment of depression but effective in handling chronic pain. The dose used to treat pain is much lower than that used to treat depression. However, it makes the dryness of the eyes and mouth worse.

The pain specialist may also use a range of other techniques; we'll look at these later in the book.

Surgery

One way to relieve dry eyes is to undergo a minor surgical procedure to seal the tear ducts that drain tears from your eyes (punctal occlusion). Collagen or silicone plugs are inserted into the ducts for a temporary closure. Collagen plugs eventually dissolve, but silicone plugs will keep the ducts sealed until they fall out or are removed. Your doctor may use a laser to permanently seal your ducts.

Medications to avoid if possible

Several types of medication can cause dryness or allergic reactions and can make your symptoms worse. Talk to your health professional if you are taking any of the following medications, but continue to take them unless advised to stop by your health professional:

- some blood pressure medications;
- antidepressants;
- anti-histamines;
- decongestants;
- diuretics;
- muscle spasm medications;
- bladder medications;
- some heart medicines;
- Parkinson's disease medications.

5

A complementary approach

Up to now, we've dealt pretty much exclusively with conventional medical approaches to Sjögren's – in other words, what you can expect if you go to see your GP or a specialist physician. Conventional medicine is very important as a means of controlling the disorder and making you more comfortable. I would never suggest abandoning it, and even though there is no cure for Sjögren's at the moment, the treatments available are the best we have.

Having said that, I do believe that there is a place for 'complementary' approaches in the treatment of Sjögren's. Non-conventional medicine and alternative therapies may not be able to cure your illness, but – used as a complement to conventional medicine – they can certainly offer relief to some.

Alternative therapies cover a huge area, from acupuncture and chiropractic to various spiritual treatments. An alternative therapy can be defined as one that is not generally taught in medical schools or used in hospitals. There are, however, exceptions. A few so-called alternative therapies, such as osteopathy, have been accepted into mainstream medicine.

Many alternative therapies imply a greater degree of involvement and responsibility on the part of the patient than is usual in conventional medicine. Another feature of alternative therapies is that many of them have not undergone any sort of rigorous scientific evaluation – though, again, there are exceptions: acupuncture, for example, has attracted several scientific studies. In many cases, however – such as homeopathy – nobody has yet managed to demonstrate why certain patients appear to recover after treatment. It is possible that certain therapies only work well on certain individuals, or with certain disorders.

Holistic medicine is frequently talked about but seldom explained. In fact, it is not just an approach to treatment but a whole philosophy. The therapist's main aim is to treat the 'whole person', taking account of not just physical symptoms but also emotional, mental and spiritual considerations.

Integrative medicine is practised by some GPs and rheumatologists. It isn't strictly one type of treatment but a dual approach that aims to blend alternative therapies with Western medicine, with the aim of finding the best in each. In this respect it is a little like holistic medicine, but it is perhaps more tolerant of conventional therapies. Practitioners of integrative medicine tend to focus on their patients as individuals, rather than on a disease or disorder in isolation.

Preventive medicine represents an important recent development, with a new emphasis from conventional medicine on keeping people well rather than just trying to cure them when they fall ill. This covers everything from advice on healthy eating and exercise to screening tests and immunization.

Why go alternative?

One of the good things about alternative therapies is that they enable patients to get involved in their own treatment. You don't get that helpless feeling you get sometimes in a consultant's clinic, when you don't really understand what's going on but are afraid to ask. Instead, you are made to feel that you have a vital part to play in your own recovery – and that is a real boost to the morale.

An improvement in morale can lead to a generally sunnier outlook on life, which can lead in turn to a reduction in perceived pain (see Chapter 6, on pain management, for more about this).

Again, I must stress that alternative therapies aren't going to cure your Sjögren's, but there may well be a treatment out there that can reduce your symptoms – physical and emotional.

Alternative medicine is not recommended as a first-line treatment for acute flare-ups, either. You may find that something like a therapeutic massage or a paraffin-wax hand bath is soothing, but when symptoms are serious and pain is more than just bothersome, do stick with conventional treatments.

Things you need to consider

If you want to experiment with complementary therapies, it is best to be as well prepared as possible. This means getting lots of information about different therapies, and finding out how much it is likely to cost you. The price per treatment session needs to be weighed against the number of sessions you are going to need. It is very easy to be talked into committing yourself to a lengthy and expensive programme of treatment without any guarantee of benefit.

Do talk to other people, particularly other people with Sjögren's, about their experiences of alternative therapy. Don't necessarily take one bad experience as a sign not to try that therapy, but equally, don't think that one alleged 'miracle cure' means that a particular therapy is some kind of universal panacea.

Do your research on the therapists; if they are reputable, they won't mind your asking about their qualifications and experience. If their profession is regulated, do they have a certificate or licence to practise? Where did they study and for how long? How long have they been practising? Again, if possible talk to other people who have used these therapists.

Last but by no means least, talk to your doctor. First of all, make sure that you have a correct diagnosis of Sjögren's. If you aren't sure what you're suffering from, it's going to be very hard to treat it! Next, talk to your GP and/or specialist about the therapy or therapies you are thinking of trying. Many doctors nowadays are open to complementary medicine, and are willing to give advice on possible benefits and/or side-effects. Even if they are not well disposed to alternative therapy, they will be able to suggest whether or not the particular treatment could interact with the medication you are taking.

If your therapist asks for a letter of referral from your GP (some GPs who are also alternative practitioners do this) and your doctor will not comply, ask why not. If after this you are still keen to try the therapy, approach another doctor in your GP practice.

Supplements

Vitamins and minerals

You may be tempted to try treating your Sjögren's with supplements, though this is still something of a lottery. What works for one person may do nothing for another, and then there is the possibility of a placebo effect. Not to mention the cost . . .

A study of people with Sjögren's by Dr Gloria Gilbère of the Naturopathic Health and Research Center, Bonners Ferry, Idaho, USA, found that many of them were deficient in zinc, as well as vitamin A, vitamin B6, potassium and calcium. Generally, however, not much information is available on how specific vitamin or mineral supplements may help in Sjögren's syndrome, though a daily multi-vitamin may be worthwhile, especially if you do tend to limit your diet due to mouth discomfort.

This said, you might like to consider the following (I'm listing food sources as well, as many experts believe vitamins are much more effective when taken as part of your usual diet):

- Vitamin C protects against inflammation and infection, and may help protect against dental caries. Chewable vitamin C is highly acidic and may damage tooth enamel, so is best avoided. Good sources are citrus fruits, berries, tomatoes, cauliflower, potatoes, green leafy vegetables, peppers.
- Vitamin B6 helps with the central nervous system and good skin condition. It's probably best taken as part of a vitamin B6 compound to avoid creating imbalances with the other B vitamins. Good food sources are fish, bananas, chicken, pork, wholegrains and dried beans.
- Riboflavin (vitamin B2) may offer relief to people who feel as if grit or sand is irritating the inside of the eyelid. B2 helps with growth, skin, nails, hair, sensitive lips and tongue and eyesight, and lack of it causes itching and irritation of the eyes, lips and skin. Good sources include milk, liver, yeast, cheese, green leafy vegetables and fish.
- Vitamin E is a good lubricant, and in oil form (some capsules contain oil) can be used around the nose, inside the nose and inside the mouth. It's found in wheatgerm, soya beans, vegetable oils, broccoli, leafy green vegetables, wholegrains, peanuts and eggs.
- Zinc may help with the decreased taste and smell suffered by some people with Sjögren's. Good sources include oysters, offal, meat, mushrooms, eggs, wholegrain products (including cereals such as porridge or branded wholegrain cereals) and brewer's yeast.
- Vitamin A has been used by some people. As severe vitamin A deficiency can cause dry eyes, some people have tried treating their Sjögren's with different forms of this vitamin, such as beta-carotene, a non-toxic form of vitamin A. Some have also reported beneficial effects from Vitamin A eye-drops. However, medical authorities caution that the dryness caused by vitamin A deficiency is different from the dry eyes that are such a feature of

Sjögren's syndrome, so it is questionable whether this sort of supplementation is really beneficial. As too much vitamin A can cause liver damage, it may be best to try and eat foods rich in vitamin A instead, such as fish-liver oil, carrots, green leafy vegetables, egg yolks, enriched margarine, milk products and yellow fruits.

- Potassium – good sources include fresh fruit and vegetables, especially bananas, dried apricots, pulses, mushrooms, potatoes and spinach.
- Calcium is found in milk and dairy products, dark green leafy vegetables, canned fish such as salmon and sardines if you eat the bones, nuts and seeds (almonds, brazils, sesame seeds), tofu, dried fruit, flour and bread, most of which is fortified with calcium, and hard water.

Other supplements

Again, this is an under-researched area where individual trial and error is probably needed before you find a supplement that suits.

- Among supplements recommended for fatigue are coenzyme Q10, L-carnitine and green barley.
- The herb goldenseal (*Hydrastis canadensis*) can be used as an antibacterial mouthwash. Use 30 drops of goldenseal, dissolved in 2 fl oz of warm water and swished about in the mouth, to help get rid of bacteria.
- Homeopathic remedies, such as nutmeg (*Nux moschata*), barberry (*Berberis vulgaris*) and hops (*Bryonia*), have been recommended for individuals with dry mouth. Try one at a time.
- According to ethnobiologist and author James Duke (*Handbook of Medicinal Spices*, Opamp Technical Books, Los Angeles, 2002), multiflora rose (*Rosa multiflora*) is used in China to moisten a dry mouth. A tea may be made from 2–4 tsp of multiflora rose, added to a cup of boiling water.
- Dr Duke also suggests consuming red pepper (capsicum) to stimulate salivation and tears. Use with discretion in cooking, not raw and alone!

What to consider when choosing a supplement

- How long will you have to take it before you can expect to experience some benefit?
- Is it likely to interact adversely with your prescribed medication?

If so, please do not try it without first consulting your doctor. And don't come off your usual medication without your doctor's agreement. Your doctor may also be able to advise about dosages.

- Are there any known side-effects or dangers?
- Do you know any other people with Sjögren's who have tried it, and did it seem to do them any good?
- Don't buy anything unless it is made by a reputable manufacturer (buying supplements on the Internet, for example, is a risky business). It might not be the real thing, it might be adulterated, and at best it may be a different strength from that stated on the bottle.
- Ideally, don't take more than one supplement at a time. And if you do, check with your doctor that the combination is safe. Just because something is advertised as 'natural' does not mean it cannot also be potent and dangerous!
- Don't take anything unless you're satisfied that it's safe – particularly if you have some other medical condition (e.g. diabetes, heart problems) that might complicate matters, or if you are pregnant (or intending to be).

Supplements – uses and possible problem areas

Here is a list of supplements that have been used by those with Sjögren's, together with their possible side-effects and drug interactions.

Bromelain	May increase effects of blood-thinning drugs and tetracycline antibiotics.
Echinacea	May counteract immune-suppressant drugs such as glucocorticoids taken for lupus and rheumatoid arthritis. May increase side-effects of methotrexate.
Evening primrose oil	Can counteract the effects of anti-convulsant drugs.
Fish oil	May increase effects of blood-thinning drugs and herbs.
Folic acid	Interferes with methotrexate; ask your doctor how to take it.
Gamma-linolenic acid (GLA)	May increase effects of blood-thinning drugs and herbs.
Garlic	Can increase effects of blood-thinning drugs and herbs.

Ginger	Can increase NSAID side-effects and effects of blood-thinning drugs and herbs.
Ginkgo	May increase effects of blood-thinning drugs and herbs.
Ginseng	May increase effects of blood-thinning drugs, oestrogens and glucocorticoids; shouldn't be used by those with diabetes; may interact with MAO inhibitors (used in certain antidepressants).
Kava kava	Can increase effects of alcohol, sedatives and tranquillizers.
Magnesium	May interact with blood-pressure medications.
St John's Wort	May enhance effects of narcotics, alcohol and antidepressants; may increase risk of sunburn; may interfere with iron absorption.
Valerian	Can increase the effects of sedatives and tranquillizers.
Zinc	Can interfere with glucocorticoids and other immunosuppressing drugs.

Glucosamine and chondroitin sulphate

Glucosamine and chondroitin sulphate are supplements frequently taken by arthritis sufferers to relieve their symptoms, and are regarded by many as 'natural' because they are substances that occur naturally in the human body. The pain relief gained is said to be similar to that obtained by taking the milder NSAIDs, such as ibuprofen and aspirin.

Glucosamine is believed to help with the repair of cartilage, while chondroitin sulphate helps to increase its elasticity. Most users find that they experience full benefit within a few months – so if it hasn't helped you by then, it probably won't.

Possible problems

- Although both products are 'natural', it is important to note that they are extracted from animal tissue. Those with shellfish allergies should beware of glucosamine, as it is extracted from crab, shrimp and lobster shells.
- Side-effects may include loose stools and flatulence.

- Pregnant women and those intending to become pregnant shouldn't use these supplements.
- Diabetics who are taking glucosamine need to check their blood sugar more frequently.
- Chondroitin sulphate may thin the blood – an important consideration for anyone using a blood-thinning drug like heparin, warfarin or daily aspirin.

Other alternative treatments

Acupuncture

Some studies suggest that acupuncture might offer some improvement in dry eyes and dry mouth symptoms. A Swedish study found that salivary flow showed significant improvement in people with dry mouth after six months of acupuncture treatment. The study recommended that, like other forms of alternative medicine, acupuncture is best used as a complement to conventional treatment.

LongoVital

A Danish study at Bispebjerg Hospital, Copenhagen, looked at whether saliva could be increased by taking LongoVital, a herbal supplement enriched with the recommended daily doses of vitamins. The research concluded that the tablet could have a beneficial and prolonged effect on saliva flow.

Evening primrose oil

There has been some speculation that evening primrose oil may help those with Sjögren's syndrome, as it provides a source of omega-3 fatty acids which could help relieve both the inflammation of Sjögren's syndrome and dry eyes.

Several trials which looked at the role of gamma-linolenic acid (GLA) in the form of evening primrose oil in primary Sjögren's syndrome have had positive results (though one other trial found no real improvement). It appears that evening primrose oil acts by correcting imbalances in the immune system, boosting activity in the saliva and tear glands, and increasing PGE1, a beneficial prostaglandin. The benefits of evening primrose oil may take several months to become noticeable.

6

Managing flare-ups and pain

Everybody has flare-ups, even if they function well most of the time or if medication usually controls their illness. They don't mean you're a failure! In fact, flare-ups can serve a purpose – however unwelcome – in signalling that your body has had enough for the moment, and needs some time out. The trick is to try and catch yourself before you reach the 'flare' point. Do try to get to know your own particular 'warning signs' – perhaps sudden increased fatigue, achiness, depression, irritability or just a feeling of being under the weather. Try and take extra rest before it becomes a problem.

Taking care of yourself and pacing yourself will help to cut down the number of flare-ups you have. Try and identify individual causes that contribute to flare-ups. Yours may vary, but common ones include:

- stress;
- fatigue;
- overwork;
- changes in routine;
- certain foods.

It may help to keep a diary for a while so that you can spot the warning signs that may precede a flare-up.

Kimberley found that, with care, she could lead a normal if sedate life. However, she had a tendency to speed up and take on too much when she felt well, and would pay heavily for this at times, becoming immobilized with fatigue and joint pain for two or three days, especially in her elbows, feet, knees and neck. Her warning sign was irritation with her children and with shop assistants! She gradually learned to pay attention to her body's messages before reaching this point, and to take more rest along the way.

Laura would have regular flare-ups once a month associated with pre-menstrual syndrome. Her eyes would become drier, she would feel cold, shivery and 'fluey', and she felt generally miserable, wanting only to huddle up in bed with a hot-water bottle. She was extremely thirsty and drank – and retained – a great deal of fluid, making her gain several pounds which she lost once her period began. Her other symptoms also eased off during the first two days of her period.

Julia worked from home and so could control her routine to a large extent. She swam three times a week – gently – and generally had a good balance of work and rest. However, she found that eating too much wheat and dairy (she loved pasta and French bread) and not enough fresh produce, combined with stress, would result in her becoming exhausted. Constipation was another warning sign, due to too much refined flour and not enough fibrous fresh stuff and fluid. She would also have a return of symptoms such as sore mouth and eyes. Then it would be time to have a complete break, and to re-stock the cupboard and fridge with fruit, vegetables and so on.

What to do if you have a flare-up: action plan

Drawing up an action plan can help minimize the distress of a flare-up even if you can't totally prevent it. You may find it helpful to stock up with what you need to help deal with flare-ups, such as medication, hot and cold packs, pillows, artificial tears and saliva, and pain-relieving gel if you find it useful.

If a flare-up strikes

- *Deal with the pain.* Have some tried-and-tested remedies for alleviating pain, whether that's via medication, a hot-water bottle, a warm bath or shower, or simply lying in bed. Warm compresses or heating pads can help ease joint or gland pain. Be careful not to use pain-relieving gel at the same time as taking NSAIDs by mouth, or you may accidentally overdose.
- *Get comfortable.* Call a halt to all activity as far as is feasible, and just rest. Use whatever simple comfort remedies suit you best, such as sucking ice cubes or frozen grapes to help reduce the pain of a dry, cracked mouth (see Chapter 3).
- *Minimize stress.* Now is not the time to engage in a tussle with the bank, to undertake the weekly shop or to invite your in-laws round. Be kind to yourself and quietly avoid as many sources of stress as possible.
- *Inform your employer.* Employers vary in how understanding they

are towards a person with chronic sickness, but ideally you should try and ensure that your employer is as well informed as possible about your condition.

- *Get the family to rally round.* Without making a huge fuss, many Sjögren's people appreciate it if the family can take over when a flare-up strikes, giving help with everyday tasks such as washing up, laundry, shopping and so on.
- *Look at your balance of exercise and rest.* As we've already discussed, you need to maintain your fitness, but you also need to recharge your batteries. If flare-ups are frequent, are you doing too much? Gentle exercise, several times a day, is far better for you than infrequent bursts of over-activity, which are more likely to prompt another flare-up.
- *Look at your balance of work and leisure.* If you are having frequent flare-ups, could a change of hours or even of jobs help? Easier said than done, I know, but maybe worthy of consideration if you feel you are having more than your fair share of flare-ups!

Managing pain

Joint pain is a recognized symptom of Sjögren's, while a few unlucky sufferers sometimes feel aches and pains throughout the entire body. Other people's experience may be more idiosyncratic – one Finnish study looked at foot pain as a symptom of Sjögren's!

However, many people with full-blown Sjögren's are also holding down demanding jobs and living a full life on top of that, with pain – if any – limited to the mild discomfort of slightly dry eyes or a shortage of saliva. An American study, from the National Institutes of Health, Bethesda, Maryland, found that only a minority of people (7 per cent) suffered widespread pain due to Sjögren's. Other people may lead a full life most of the time but be swamped by profound fatigue and/or aches and pains if they overreach their personal limits and try and do too much. Still others may experience pain, which may be mild and short-term or more severe and more persistent. So, because each person will have an individual experience of his or her disease, any therapies will need to be tailored to particular problems.

From a physical perspective, having pain in a certain part of the body often makes people reluctant to use that particular joint or group of muscles. As a result, they end up suffering from muscle weakness and bad posture – which, of course, cause further discomfort. A loss of muscle tone and overall lack of fitness is a major factor in chronic pain, so improving your general physical condition can make a big difference to the way you feel. Exercise is also well known to boost production of endorphins, the body's natural pain-relieving hormones. (See Chapter 8 for more on exercise.)

The pain mechanism

Pain is the body's response to an unpleasant stimulus. When you bang your head or burn your finger, specialized nerve endings detect what is happening and relay pain messages to the peripheral nervous system. This in turn sends messages along the nerve pathways to the central nervous system (the spinal cord and brain).

Scientific research suggests that these pain signals have to reach a threshold before they are relayed. This is known as the 'pain gate' theory, as it is as if a certain level of signal opens a gate, letting the pain through. It is only when the gate is open that we feel pain. Modern pain clinics can teach patients ways of closing the gate and reducing the pain they experience.

After the unpleasant stimulus has gone, a part of the brain called the thalamus should send out a signal telling the pain to stop. Most of the time this happens, but sometimes the system goes wrong and the pain persists as chronic pain.

Within the brain and nervous system, certain chemicals called neurotransmitters are produced. Some kinds of neurotransmitters – for example serotonin and norepinephrine – seem to be able to decrease pain signals by making the pain sensors release endorphins, the body's natural painkillers.

Although we tend to think of pain as a purely physical thing, in reality it is closely bound up with our psychological wellbeing. If you are depressed, for instance, you are likely to feel greater pain than if you are optimistic and happy. People who have been brought up to ignore pain as much as possible generally feel it less intensely than those who associate pain with great distress and suffering.

So, if we want to reduce the amount of pain we feel, we need to:

- get the body to produce more endorphins;
- think positive.

Different types of pain

As we've seen, there is more than one kind of pain. In fact, there are three main types:

Acute

This kind of pain is temporary, and lessens as an injury heals or a condition abates. It is generally directly related to tissue damage.

Chronic malignant

This is the pain experienced by people suffering from various forms of cancer.

Chronic non-malignant

This is pain that persists, even after a flare-up has died down – and it is common among sufferers from Sjögren's and fibromyalgia. Somehow, the nervous system stops acting normally and starts generating nothing but pain, even though no further damage is being done to the body. This has been described as a sort of memory of pain. It has no purpose, as it is not protecting the body.

Some chronic pain results from damage to nerve fibres, for example after an attack of shingles, and is called neuropathic pain. Again, these damaged nerves persist in sending out pain messages even though there is no continuing tissue damage.

Chronic pain can range from mild to agonizing and very disabling. Even if it is not severe, the fact that it is there all the time can wreak havoc with sufferers' lives, leading to a feeling of loss of control. This in turn leads to depression, which leads to more pain. It is important to treat acute pain quickly and effectively, or there is a danger that it may develop into chronic pain.

Help from your doctor

If you suffer chronic or long-term pain, you may well need professional help. The first thing is to establish *why* the pain is present. The approach to eye discomfort due to lack of tears is very different from the approach to the widespread muscle pains experienced by those unfortunate enough to have a combination of Sjögren's and fibromyalgia.

So, do see your doctor if you are experiencing pain which you can't control by your own efforts. Doctors are better than ever before at controlling pain and helping people regain control of their lives, and this may be particularly relevant if you also suffer from another or associated condition such as arthritis or fibromyalgia. For many patients with Sjögren's syndrome it is the fatigue rather than pain which is the major problem. For others, however, pain may be the dominant problem, particularly if features of fibromyalgia are also present. This is notoriously difficult to treat and specialist pain clinics may help.

Depending on which facilities are available locally, your family doctor may be able to refer you to someone who specializes in pain management if your case is severe.

Some areas may have access to a specialist pain clinic, with a multidisciplinary approach to treating pain, or a local GP with a special interest in pain relief. Many pain consultants are anaesthetists, who have a comprehensive knowledge of all methods of pain control, from medication to physiotherapy, nerve blocks to acupuncture. Other professionals may be involved from a range of disciplines – including alternative therapies – such as physiotherapy, occupational therapy, clinical psychology, counselling, relaxation therapy, specialist nursing, acupuncture.

Clinical psychologists are often included because, as mentioned earlier, the perception of pain is strongly influenced by your state of mind.

Pain management programmes can help with long-term problems of chronic pain, and aim to break the cycle of pain, loss of fitness, and depression. You can be referred to a pain management programme either by your GP or by a pain clinic.

As with the pain clinic, sessions are taught by a multidisciplinary team made up of doctors, nurses, physiotherapists, occupational therapists, clinical psychologists and pain specialists. It is worth looking at the topics they cover because many of them can be practised in your own home:

- *Relaxation techniques*: it is surprisingly easy to learn how to relax, using swiftly taught techniques. Relaxation reduces muscle tension and anxiety, and helps to ease pain. (See Chapter 7 for more on relaxation.)
- *Occupational therapy*: this deals with finding practical ways of doing daily tasks which you may currently find difficult or impossible (e.g. household activities such as ironing, mowing the lawn, vacuuming). This helps you to gradually get back into life

and work, increasing morale and reducing pain. Occupational therapists will also emphasize the importance of pacing yourself. If you do too much one day, you will pay for it with pain the next. Far better to ration the amount you do per day – you will probably get more done in the long run.

- *Physiotherapy and exercise*: even though you may think you are incapable of staggering down the road to the post office, you can learn the benefits of stretching, strengthening and aerobic exercise. And you will soon realize that – with care and determination – anyone can exercise: even me! Slow stretches relax muscles and ease tension, and low-impact exercise like walking, swimming and cycling is ideal for building up strength, general fitness and flexibility. Don't forget that exercise helps to release those pain-relieving endorphins too! The golden rule is: don't do too much, too quickly. Ease into it gradually, or you may do more harm than good. (See Chapter 8 for more on exercise.)

- *Family therapy/counselling*: some courses include a session for partners and other family members, to help increase their understanding and ease relationship problems. And, of course, we mustn't forget the benefits of just being in a room, talking to other people. When the course finishes, you can continue the benefits by having follow-up meetings, joining a support group such as the British Sjögren's Syndrome Association (BSSA; see Useful Addresses, p. 90) or becoming involved in online discussion forums (again, see Useful Addresses).

Medication

Medication, while important, is not always the be-all and end-all of pain control and stronger medication may not control your pain more effectively than a less strong drug.

Timing is important, and most drugs need to be taken at set intervals for maximum effectiveness. It may be that regular, moderate doses of a medium-strength analgesic are more useful in controlling your pain than less well-timed doses of stronger medication.

Pain clinics use a wide variety of pills and potions. Not all of them were designed originally as pain-relieving drugs.

NSAIDs	Non-steroidal anti-inflammatories. Over-the-counter varieties include ibuprofen and aspirin.
Paracetamol (acetaminophen)	Good at controlling pain and fever, but less effective at combating inflammation.
Narcotics	Generally the last resort in terms of analgesia. Although recent research suggests that drugs like morphine are not necessarily addictive when used to combat pain, doctors are still reluctant to prescribe them except in cases of terminal illness.
Antidepressants	It has been shown that older types of antidepressant, such as amitriptyline, can be useful in treating chronic pain. They are non-addictive, but do have side-effects, such as increasing dryness in the mouth (not good for those with Sjögren's!) and constipation.
Anticonvulsants	Some drugs originally designed for the treatment of epilepsy, e.g. gabapentin and carbamazepine, have been proven to be effective in treating chronic nerve pain.
Corticosteroids	Drugs like prednisolone are very good at reducing inflammation and swelling, but (as seen earlier) they do have potentially serious side-effects.
Tramadol	This is a synthetic analgesic, used mainly for chronic pain but also sometimes to treat acute pain.
Capsaicin	This is not an oral drug but a topical cream derived from chilli peppers. Not surprisingly, when it is applied to the skin there is an initial burning sensation. It is believed to work by interrupting pain signals.

7
How to help yourself –
lifestyle issues

Being involved in your own care is really important in Sjögren's syndrome. Experts believe it can make a real difference to your overall wellbeing and quality of life, and just taking some measure of control is well demonstrated to have a beneficial effect in most conditions. Besides, with a condition like Sjögren's, which has such a variety of symptoms, being involved yourself is often the most effective way of dealing with those symptoms. This chapter looks at lifestyle issues that can help, such as getting plenty of rest, eating well and doing mild exercise daily.

Fatigue

Tiredness is probably the leading complaint in people with Sjögren's syndrome. This may have more than one cause, depending on whether or not you have another condition as well as Sjögren's, and can also take different forms.

Some experts describe two sorts of fatigue in Sjögren's syndrome:

- *Late morning or early afternoon fatigue*, when you get up full of energy but tend to 'run out of steam' later in the day. This is sometimes called 'inflammatory fatigue'. People suffering this tend to report flu-like symptoms.
- *Morning fatigue*, when you get up feeling you have not had a proper night's rest because your sleep has been disrupted. This is also quite common in both Sjögren's syndrome and fibromyalgia. There may be specific causes, such as joint or muscle pain, which can disrupt sleep. Another common cause of sleep disruption is having to get up frequently in the night in order to go to the bathroom – a result of fluid intake during the day because of dry mouth and throat. Obviously, it makes sense to tackle the specific symptoms here – for example, sucking on ice chips during the day instead of taking long drinks of water; or using humidifiers and oral lubricants (i.e. saliva substitutes) to avoid drinking altogether.

Tips to increase your energy

• Listen to your body and do take rest when you need it. Try alternating rest with exercise. Gradually increasing your exercise may also help decrease your fatigue.

• Talk to your doctor about any medications that might contribute to fatigue, such as tranquillizers. However, be sure to continue to take any medications prescribed for Sjögren's syndrome unless your doctor feels they should be discontinued, and then do follow carefully any directions for withdrawal. Never abruptly discontinue a medication without medical advice.

• Don't skip meals, especially breakfast. Bear in mind that improving your diet generally may increase your energy level.

• Reduce your use of caffeine, nicotine, sugary foods and alcohol, which tend to contribute to fatigue.

• Cut back on watching television, and instead spend time with friends, try new activities or travel to break the fatigue cycle.

• Bear in mind that tiredness may be related to another health problem, such as thyroid problems or depression. Do consult your doctor if fatigue persists despite your best endeavours.

• Some people find they actually need a rest in bed in the early afternoon and are then able to get going again.

Getting a good night's sleep

Whatever the reasons for poor sleep, it is important not to let them become ingrained. Once you have tackled any underlying causes such as excessive urination, it can be very helpful to establish a good sleep pattern as follows:

• Stick to the same bedtime and also try to get up at the same time each morning. Try not to oversleep no matter how poorly you have slept the night before.

• If you can't sleep, sit in bed and undertake a restful activity such as reading, knitting or doing a puzzle. This takes the pressure off you to get to sleep.

• Ensure you have enough daily exercise, but avoid exercise in the evening as it can leave you too stimulated to sleep.

• Try stress reduction techniques such as meditation, biofeedback or progressive relaxation.

• Avoid caffeine after lunch, and alcohol after dinner, or cut them out altogether. In some people, even one cup of coffee or one alcoholic drink is enough to disturb sleep.

- The bedroom should be quiet, dark and comfortable. Don't use it for work – try and create a restful association with sleep in this room.
- During the daytime, try and get at least one hour of natural light, as some evidence shows it can strengthen circadian rhythms and improve the quality of sleep.
- Sometimes following good sleep habits is not enough to improve the sense of daytime fatigue and poor sleep. In this case, do consult your doctor about possible specific sleep disorders, such as sleep apnoea, when breathing is interrupted during sleep. Snoring, or waking gasping for breath, can be a sign of sleep apnoea, which can be a risk in cases of recent weight gain – often a side-effect of corticosteroids. This requires specialist evaluation and treatment so your doctor may refer you to a sleep expert.

Making your bed comfortable

Some people with Sjögren's find it helps to make minor changes to their bed – though you may remember Mandy, from Chapter 1, who made her husband go out and buy her a new mattress only to find that her aches and pains were just as bad! However, at this point Mandy hadn't been diagnosed with Sjögren's and didn't realize she had it – with this kind of illness, it is very much finding out about what helps you as an individual. For some, a new mattress may indeed help!

- To take the weight off painful feet and ankles, try fitting a cradle towards the lower end of the bed to lift bedclothes off your lower limbs.
- If you spend long periods in bed, a board beneath the mattress will provide extra support for your back.
- A board laid across the bottom half of the mattress will enable you to walk your feet back and forth under the cradle while lying down, as gentle exercise.
- A slant-board, which gently tilts you head-down in the bed, can help circulation as well as relieving the joints from the pressure of gravity – though if you suffer from reflux you may prefer to raise the head of your bed by a few inches.

Not forgetting sex

At a time when Sjögren's syndrome may be attacking your lifestyle and identity, loss of intimacy can be particularly upsetting. Some people feel too exhausted or unwell for much physical contact, but may feel they're missing out emotionally, especially as time goes on. And of course the implications for a relationship may need to be addressed. To some people, sex may seem like a minor issue, but it does help you to maintain closeness with your partner.

- Aim for effective pain control – look at the advice in Chapter 6 on managing pain, and consult your doctor about medication.
- Alleviate vaginal dryness with artificial lubricants (see the advice on this in Chapter 3).
- Don't underestimate tiredness as a cause of lost desire – have a look at the suggestions for beating fatigue in this chapter.
- Try and ensure that your diet is as good as possible – again, look at the section on diet in this chapter, and also consider the advice on supplements in Chapter 5.
- Do consult your doctor if you fear you may be anaemic – again, fatigue from anaemia can kill interest in close contact.
- If you don't feel up to sex, don't minimize the importance of a good cuddle!

Diet

A healthy diet is part of taking care of yourself under any circumstances, and is doubly important if you have Sjögren's, though it may need some thought and adjustment. A sore, dry mouth, possible gingivitis and tooth problems may all contribute to make a normal diet less appetizing – yet now is the time when you need to obtain the maximum nutrients from your food.

Generally, you may find you get on better with moister, more fluid foods – soups, casseroles, mousses, smoothies and the like. Such foods may take a little more preparation but are worth the extra effort if you are using fresh ingredients. A better diet will result in better health and improved energy levels.

Try and avoid alcoholic drinks and caffeine, which are dehydrating and can contribute to increased dryness. Spicy and acidic food can also irritate your mouth, and sugary food can promote further tooth decay.

The lack of saliva has important implications, and any foods likely to erode tooth enamel should be avoided, such as sugary drinks, alcohol and citrus fruits like lemons. Hot and spicy foods may also need to be cut out or limited, such as curries, foods containing chilli, and some fast and packaged foods that can be hard on the moisture-producing glands.

Some people have found that they react badly to the food additive monosodium glutamate, the artificial sweetener aspartame (Nutra-sweet) and the preservative citric acid (which causes mouth sores in some), and that Sjögren's symptoms diminish when they avoid these food substances.

A high intake of calcium, in dairy products such as milk, cheese and yoghurt, will help boost tooth health. Plain live yoghurt may also help prevent thrush in the mouth. Some people with Sjögren's develop lactose intolerance, so if you cannot tolerate dairy products look for other good sources of calcium such as dark green leafy vegetables, sesame seeds, canned fish if you eat the bones, hard water, dried figs, bread and the humble baked bean!

Essential fatty acids (EFAs)

Found in several fish and vegetable oils, EFAs play a vital role in good heart health as well as promoting the smooth running of the immune and nervous systems. In an auto-immune condition such as Sjögren's they are therefore vitally important.

We need EFAs to manufacture and repair cell membranes, and to produce prostaglandins, which regulate body functions such as heart rate, blood pressure, blood clotting, fertility and conception, and play a role in immune function by regulating inflammation and encouraging the body to fight infection. Lack of EFAs has been linked with several health conditions, including heart disease and cancer as well as other auto-immune disorders such as lupus and rheumatoid arthritis. There is some evidence that EFAs help reduce inflammation, which can be a feature of Sjögren's.

Omega 6

Omega 6, or linolenic acid, is found in:

- vegetables;
- fruits;
- nuts;
- grains;

- seeds;
- oils made from safflower, sunflower, corn, soya, evening primrose, pumpkin and wheatgerm.

Omega 3

Omega 3, or alpha-linolenic acid, is found in:

- fish oil – though flaxseed oil (see below) contains twice as much as is found in fish oil!
- flaxseeds (linseeds);
- mustard seeds;
- pumpkin seeds;
- soya beans;
- walnut oil;
- green leafy vegetables;
- grains;
- spirulina;
- oils made from linseed (flaxseeds), rapeseed (canola) or soya beans. One tablespoon a day of flaxseed oil should provide the recommended daily adult portion of linolenic acid.

How to make the best of EFAs

High heat, light and oxygen destroy EFAs, so when consuming foods for their EFA content try to avoid cooked or heated forms. For example, raw nuts are a better source than roasted nuts. Don't use flaxseed oil for cooking, and never re-use any type of oil. Extra virgin olive oil or grapeseed oil are best to use for cooking oil, as they withstand high heat well.

Replace hydrogenated fats (like margarine), cholesterol-based fats (butter/dairy products) and polysaturated fats (common cooking oils) with healthy EFA-based fats when possible. For example, instead of margarine or butter on your vegetables, use flaxseed and/or extra virgin olive oils.

Another idea is to grind flaxseed to sprinkle on vegetables for a slightly nutty taste. Whole flaxseeds are usually passed through the intestine, simply absorbing water and not yielding much oil.

Swallowing problems

As already explained, some people with Sjögren's have problems swallowing. In this case, it can be all too easy to limit your choice of foods to what is easiest or most convenient, so ending up with an inadequate diet. To maximize the benefits from your food choices, consider the following:

- Make the most of soups using a blender – meat, vegetables, lentils, soya beans and other beans and legumes can all be pureed to make nourishing liquid meals.
- Add eggs, cheese, tofu or dry skimmed-milk powder to increase protein.
- Casseroles can also be good. Cut food into bite-sized or smaller pieces (a pair of scissors is handy for meat) and add to a sauce.
- Mash or puree vegetables and fruits.
- Add interest to sauces using yoghurt, tomatoes and low-fat fromage frais.
- Consider buying a juicer to make wonderful combinations of vegetables, such as carrot and sprouted alfalfa, or of fruit, such as blueberry and banana.
- Make the most of eggs, which are nourishing and can be scrambled, poached or made into custards.
- Use jellies, ice creams, custards, and milk shakes and smoothies. Adding silken tofu to these will boost protein.
- Eat a number of small meals or snacks a day, rather than one or two big ones.
- Rinse your mouth regularly to remove debris, add freshness and lubricate your mouth.

Coping with digestive problems

Julia found she had a lot of abdominal discomfort. Eating too much wheat and dairy products in particular seemed to upset her delicate digestive balance, resulting in windy pains and bloating. She was never sure whether to connect this with her Sjögren's or with stress, or both.

Lack of moisture can affect the oesophagus and other inner digestive organs, so you may need to take some extra measures to counteract this. For example, some people with Sjögren's suffer irritable bowel syndrome too (IBS) and/or constipation, causing lower abdominal pain and alteration in bowel habit, thought to be associated with low intestinal mucous secretions. Try increasing the fibre in your diet.

To increase fibre

- Use wholegrain breads and cereals – use as croutons in soup, or as breadcrumbs to top casseroles or puddings, or as dumplings in casseroles.
- Try and eat apples and potatoes unpeeled – if you find apples sour, choose sweeter varieties and cut into small pieces.
- Make soups with dried beans or legumes.
- Add dates or figs to puddings, or make into sauces to go with ice cream.
- Make raw soups sometimes, such as uncooked tomatoes and fresh parsley, or carrot and orange juice.
- Try finely grated salads such as carrot and raisin, or red cabbage. Top salads with seeds such as sunflower, sesame or pumpkin.

Food allergy and intolerance

It has been speculated that food allergy or intolerance is implicated in Sjögren's. Unfortunately no specific tests for allergy or intolerance exist, so it is usually a matter of trial and error to find out if a particular food is disagreeing with you. Common foods that cause allergy or intolerance include milk, eggs, nuts, fish and shellfish, wheat and flour, chocolate, artificial colours, pork and bacon, chicken, tomatoes, soft fruit, cheese and yeast.

The most common symptoms of allergy include asthma, gastro-intestinal symptoms (nausea, vomiting and diarrhoea), eczema, urticaria (hives), rhinorrhea (heavy discharge from the nose) and angio-oedema (swelling of the blood vessels). Other more long-term symptoms can include depression, anxiety, fatigue, migraine and sleeplessness. Again, whether this is down to diet or to Sjögren's can be difficult to determine. If you think that excluding or limiting a food will help improve your quality of life, it may be worth a try. Take foods one at a time and allow two weeks for any effect to be made.

Heartburn

Because saliva normally plays such a major role in neutralizing stomach acid, some people with Sjögren's find they are more prone to heartburn. Antacids may help. Try also raising the head of your bed, using two or three books or wood blocks, so as to prevent gastric acid from washing back into the oesophagus at night. If your problem is severe, discuss medication with your doctor, though bear in mind that medicines containing sucralfate, designed to 'coat' the oesophagus and stomach, might actually interfere with the absorption of other medications.

Swallowing your medication

Because saliva normally helps you swallow things down, you may find that pills – especially if large – can become stuck to 'dry' walls of the oesophagus, causing pain and sometimes a feeling of choking. This can have implications if you need to take medications at regular intervals but aren't digesting them 'on time' because they are getting stuck halfway down.

Try and arrange to have coated tablets when possible. Take medication with plenty of water while sitting or standing, and don't lie down immediately afterwards.

Smoking

This one is easy – don't do it! Apart from its more widely publicized health effects, smoking is exceedingly drying and can damage your mouth, nose, eyes and lungs, so making symptoms of Sjögren's worse. In fact, few people with Sjögren's are smokers, and this may be a silver lining of the disease!

If you do need to stop, here are some suggestions to help you on your way:

• Prepare yourself for quitting; set a special day such as a birthday or anniversary.
• Read as much information on stopping smoking as you can.
• Involve a friend and get someone to stop smoking with you if possible.
• Be realistic – you will have withdrawal symptoms, but they will go away.
• Keep a diary and note when you tend to smoke and what triggers the need to light up. Then try and avoid those situations when you do smoke.
• Calculate how much money you'll save by not smoking – and plan what you could spend the money on.

- Magnesium can help reduce cravings.
- If you do relapse, be positive and consider it a learning experience. Just go back to your quitting plan. Most people have a few goes before they finally stop smoking.

Travel

There is no reason why you shouldn't travel, provided you pace yourself so it doesn't become too tiring. Listed below are a few hints that hopefully will make your journey more enjoyable.

- *Medication* – take enough medicines to last you the trip – in fact, a spare set can be useful as a back-up in case one gets lost. Have one in your hand luggage and the other packed in your suitcase.
- *Time zones* – if you're changing time zones and are on medication, do ask your doctor's advice about whether this will affect your medication.
- *Air travel* – notoriously drying, this can present special challenges to those with Sjögren's. Make sure you stay hydrated – moisten your nasal passages with a saline solution and drink plenty of water at regular intervals throughout the flight. If you do feel unwell while flying, tell a flight attendant. They are well trained and equipped for emergencies.
- *Travel sickness pills* – be careful about taking these as they may exacerbate mouth dryness.
- *Luggage* – most of us take far too much! A good general rule is to take half the amount of clothes you think you will need – the last thing you want is to exhaust yourself dragging round a heavy case. Use lightweight bags or wheeled cases, trolleys and/or a porter.

Avoiding stress

Stress definitely makes Sjögren's worse for some people. Patricia, a young mother of two, made her own list of personal de-stressors after realizing there was a direct link between how much stress she experienced and how bad her condition was. These included:

- Make no major decisions.
- Stop rushing and pace myself.
- Check what food I've been eating – and eat some fresh fruit if I've eaten a lot of junk.
- Get some sunlight or daylight.
- Change my routine.
- Play with the children.
- Talk to someone.
- Lower my expectations.
- Write down three positive statements about my life.

Richard, a rare male with Sjögren's who also suffers from lupus, says he drops everything and gets out of the house or office as soon as possible if he's feeling stressed. 'Of course, it's not always possible if I'm in a meeting, but just planning to get away for a few minutes is a big help. It gives me a feeling of control and I know that once out in the open air I forget my frustration very quickly.'

It may help to make a list of the things which cause stress in your life, and how this affects you, your family and your job. Questions to ask yourself could be:

- Is the stress short- or long-term?
- How much control do I have over it? Or do I perceive someone else to be in charge (i.e. boss, partner), and if so, how far can I accept this?
- What are my biggest obstacles to reducing stress?
- Do I have a support system of friends and/or family that will help me make positive changes?
- What am I willing to change or give up for a less stressful and tension-filled life?

Tips for reducing or controlling stress

Beating stress may take time and determination, especially if it has been persisting for a while, and if it is really severe you may also need to consider lifestyle changes. Chronic stress can sometimes be a 'wake-up' call summoning you to a change of job, a change of career, or other major shifts in your life.

We all have an individual tolerance level for stress, so, as with other aspects of Sjögren's, it is a matter of finding your own limits and doing your best to live within these limits, rather than just paying lip service to them.

There is nothing noble about enduring stressful situations, so do try and change or avoid them. If they are unavoidable, such as getting through a long working day, work out a compromise: take short breaks; go somewhere quiet for a few minutes. At home have a hot bath, sit quietly and listen to soothing music. Take time to unwind and gather your resources. If it means negotiation with an employer, do it in the confidence that compromise is a constructive solution.

- *Learn how to pace yourself* – adapting a moderate pace, keeping a regular schedule and getting adequate rest and exercise can help you better manage your illness.
- *Learn to say no* – perhaps the most important stress-management skill you can master. It's especially important to pace yourself on days when you feel energetic and may be tempted to overdo it.
- *Wait before making a decision* – bear in mind that you can take a decision after further consideration. So, a useful phrase is, 'May I come back to you on that one?' if you're not sure whether to say yes or no to an activity. Points to consider could include: can I realistically do this? Is it better to say no at the start, rather than embroiling myself and then finding I don't have the strength to finish? How much can I do? Is the deadline realistic? What adjustments can I make?
- *Don't hesitate to ask for help if you need it* – this could be help with daily chores such as washing up, or a sympathetic listening ear from a friend. But if you think that you may be under more stress than just dealing with a passing difficulty, it may be helpful to talk with your doctor, who may be able to suggest professional counselling.
- *Assess your responsibilities* – are you taking on more than you can or should handle?
- *Be realistic, not perfect* – you may expect too much of yourself and others, and then feel frustrated or let down when matters turn out less than perfectly.
- *Go easy with criticism* – of others and yourself. Try suspending all judgements for a day (including 'should', 'ought' and 'must', used of yourself). Give in occasionally, even if you think you're in the right – put your health and peace of mind first.
- *Meditate* – just ten to twenty minutes of quiet reflection may bring relief from chronic stress as well as increasing your tolerance to it.

Use the time to listen to music, relax and try to think of pleasant things or nothing.

- *Visualize* – use your imagination and picture how you can manage a stressful situation more successfully. Whether it's a business presentation or moving to a new place, many people feel visual rehearsals boost self-confidence and enable them to take a more positive approach to a difficult task.

- *Break down tasks* – do one task at a time. When you're stressed, even a normal workload can sometimes feel overwhelming, so try and take one bit of it at a time. If you feel very stressed, start with something very simple, such as putting a letter in an envelope – trivial as it sounds, any activity can help break down the feeling that you can't cope.

- *Exercise* – regular exercise is a popular way to relieve stress. Twenty to thirty minutes of physical activity two or three times a week benefits both the body and the mind.

- *Keep up hobbies* – take a break from your worries by doing something you enjoy. Whether it's gardening or painting, schedule time to indulge your interest.

- *A healthy lifestyle is key* – good nutrition makes a difference, with minimal or no caffeine and alcohol. Get enough rest, and balance exercise, work and relaxation.

Relaxation and creative visualization

These may take some practice, but they work together, not just to ease tension but to promote a more positive outlook and self-image. You can, of course, choose the images that suit you best, but a sample relaxation scenario can be as follows:

Imagine you are setting off from home. You go through a beautiful wood with a cool, clear stream running through it. There are fish swimming in the stream. You climb up a gentle slope and find a bench, where you sit for a while. You think of all the things that are worrying or hurting you, one by one, and give each one a colour and a shape. When you get up from the bench, you leave these 'objects' behind you and walk away from them.

You keep on walking through the wood until at last it opens out on to a beautiful sandy cove. The sea is washing gently on to the shore and birds are calling overhead. The sun is warm but not too hot or bright.

You find a comfortable spot and sit down, leaning back against the warm cliff-face, closing your eyes as you listen to the swish of the sea and the cries of the birds. You feel calm, untroubled, serene.

You stay there for a while and then, as afternoon is drawing on, you decide it is time to leave. You open your eyes, stand up and return home, knowing that you can come back to this place any time you close your eyes, and that when you do you will feel the same calmness again.

8

Exercise and physiotherapy

It's generally agreed that mild exercise can be beneficial for those with Sjögren's syndrome. Gentle activities such as walking or swimming can help keep joints and muscles flexible, and may also boost your energy and mood, and protect against further joint damage. But there may well be times when you feel just too exhausted to manage anything. The trick is to balance rest and activity.

To rest or not to rest?

For many people, the pain and stiffness associated with Sjögren's are often worse first thing in the morning, and the temptation is probably to do as little as possible. The same applies at times during the day, especially if you suffer so-called 'inflammatory fatigue', or late morning or early afternoon fatigue, when you may get up feeling vigorous but find your energy suddenly evaporates later on in the day.

Rest is certainly a vital part of coping with Sjögren's and it is important to listen to your body and not to push yourself too far. Don't feel guilty about taking the rest you need, especially if you have fever and fatigue. Regular rest periods can be key in helping you to pace yourself.

At the same time, it's also generally recognized that it is better for your overall physical health – and mental wellbeing – if you take regular, mild exercise. In the olden days some 30 or 40 years ago, people were sometimes taken into hospital and given bed-rest for weeks or months to help soothe inflamed joints – sometimes with limbs in splints. With too much bed-rest, unused muscles become weaker, bones lose calcium and become more brittle, and your general physical fitness declines.

Times have changed, and your doctor is now more likely to advise a nice walk or gentle swim! The balance of rest and exercise can be a fine one, but both need to be maintained in Sjögren's.

Exercise has several important functions in Sjögren's syndrome.

First, it helps maintain and maximize the mobility of any affected joints. Regular aerobic exercise builds up the resilience and capacity of the heart, lungs and circulation.

Research at the University of Missouri, Columbia, USA, found that strengthening exercises and low-impact aerobic exercise for people with arthritis resulted in improved stamina, less fatigue and an improved level of general physical functioning. As stiff and painful joints are symptoms of both arthritis and Sjögren's, the results can be taken as encouraging for people who suffer from either or both disorders.

Exercise is also well proven to improve quality of life, resulting in less muscle tension, lower stress and anxiety levels, improved energy levels, increased self-esteem and a better night's sleep. It also builds up bone strength and guards against osteoporosis.

Laura was the world's worst exerciser – until she started getting short of breath. She would puff and pant by the time she got to the top of the stairs and was thoroughly frightened that she had heart disease, asthma or some unknown complication of her Sjögren's. She felt she must have more fresh air, and started taking daily walks outside. This simple measure improved her fitness and wellbeing beyond what she could have imagined. She now manages a swim once a week or fortnight as well – not enough, she feels, but better than nothing, and a lot better than before.

Which exercise?

Individual exercise programmes vary greatly. Laura, as we saw, was keen on her daily walk; Julia was a yoga devotee; and Kimberley worked with a physiotherapist from the hospital rheumatology department on exercises designed to help her painful joints.

In general, little and often is better than long bouts of exercise. Alternating exercise and rest is also recommended, possibly combining the two: lying down while doing gentle exercise like rotating the ankles and wrists, for example.

There are different types of exercises:

• *Range-of-motion exercises* reduce stiffness and help keep your joints moving. A range-of-motion exercise for your shoulder would be to move your arm in a large circle.

- *Moderate stretching exercises* help relieve the pain and keep the muscles and tendons around an affected joint flexible and strong.
- *Strengthening exercises* maintain or increase muscle strength.
- *Endurance exercises* strengthen your heart, give you energy and keep your body flexible. These exercises include walking, swimming and cycling.

Range-of-motion and moderate stretching exercises

Range-of-motion exercises are important for those with Sjögren's, especially when the joints are inflamed during a flare-up. The goal is to reduce stiffness and minimize loss of mobility in the affected joints. They take the joint through the fullest range of movement which it can manage once or twice a day or whenever you feel the need to reduce stiffness. Pay special attention to the point at which movement becomes difficult or impossible but don't push it to the point of pain. Once the acute inflammation has died down, range-of-motion exercises become part of the warm-up to the daily exercise routine. A pattern of ten minutes warm-up, fifteen minutes work-out, five minutes cool-down is common.

Stretching is a variation on range-of-motion exercise. It involves stretching the joint to just beyond the limit of comfort, as opposed to staying just within the comfort zone. No one will tell you to stretch to the level of actual pain, and you shouldn't 'bounce' the joint in an attempt to extend it further. By putting the joint through its paces regularly, stiffness and pain are reduced. Range-of-motion exercises are even better done in water because the buoyancy of the water supports the body and protects the joints from rapid or stressful movement.

Strengthening exercises

Muscles that may have become weak through lack of use need to be rebuilt gradually by exercise. Strengthening exercises come at different levels. Isometric exercise involves clenching and unclenching muscle groups without external movement. It can be done lying or sitting down and should be part of the exercise routine even when the joints are seriously inflamed, to minimize the weakening of muscles from disuse. Isotonic exercises involve contracting the muscle and moving the joint – for example, in lifting weights.

Isometric strengthening exercises introduce an external pressure point and can probably be used after a flare-up when inflammation has died down. For example, you might push against a sofa, tightening your arm muscles but without moving wrists, elbows or shoulders. But don't try push-ups, which involve lifting the body's weight and can be too much of a strain.

Endurance exercises

Just as your leg and arm muscles become weak with disuse, so do the heart, lungs and blood vessels if not made to work. Cardiovascular exercise (the 'cardio' bit relates to the heart, 'vascular' refers to the blood vessels, and lung function is also involved) is important for general fitness and increases the capacity of the heart, lungs and blood vessels to work efficiently under stress by using oxygen efficiently.

The best kind of cardiovascular exercise for someone with Sjögren's will involve moderate effort but no jolting of joints (as in jumping – impact exercise), so try swimming (breast-stroke rather than crawl if the shoulders are affected), walking, cycling, climbing up and down stairs (unless the knees are still inflamed).

Depending on the joints affected, some form of low-impact aerobic exercise – like patting a ball against the wall or dancing (waltz, not salsa) – may also be attempted once the inflammation is in retreat. Once the muscles show signs of regaining strength and supporting affected joints adequately, it may be possible to start working with weights, under professional guidance.

Don't overdo it

You may have heard exercise fanatics talk about 'feeling the burn'. However, 'no pain, no gain' is not the case here! It's probably good if you aim to be a little bit breathless after exercise – this shows that the activity has increased your heart rate and so improved your cardiovascular performance and stamina. However, do take heed of any warning signs such as pain, shortness of breath after exercise, prolonged fatigue, dizziness, chest pain or increased joint pain – and stop. Don't push your body.

Build up a routine gradually – start with just five minutes at a time, or with three or four gentle stretches or yoga positions. Then try building up to ten to fifteen minutes three times a day, and increasing this to half an hour's exercise several times a week.

Do remember you are doing this to keep as fit and healthy as possible, not to compete as a professional athlete. If you find yourself suffering, stop.

How to get the most from your exercise

Walking, swimming and cycling are three excellent ways to get the exercise you need. Depending on your state of health and circumstances, you'll probably find that one suits you better than the others. For example, if you suffer from painful leg joints or extreme fatigue, you may prefer cycling or swimming to walking.

Walking

- Warm up for walking by doing range-of-motion exercises for knees and hips.
- Soak your feet in warm water and do range-of-motion foot exercises.
- Wear supportive walking shoes or athletic sneakers with good shock-absorbers.
- Walk on the flat where possible (beside a river); avoid hills.
- Swing your arms for balance while walking.
- If your feet feel warm after walking, soak them in cool water afterwards.

Cycling

- Adjust the seat height of your saddle so that your legs are fully straightened when pedalling.
- Set the handlebars so that they are not too low or far away from the saddle. A prone position puts strain on the lower back, shoulders, elbows and wrists.
- Adjust the pedal tension to the lowest level to limit strain on the knees.
- If the weather is bad try an indoor exercise bike.
- If your knees get painful try an indoor bike with arm motion attachments.
- Cool down with light pedalling as a substitute for range-of-motion exercises.

Swimming

- If possible, do a training session under the guidance of a trained physiotherapist.
- Breathe regularly from your diaphragm during exercise.

- Check the temperature of the pool before swimming. Temperatures between 28 and 30°C (82 and 86°F) are best for aerobic exercise. Higher than this increases vasodilatation and may make you feel light-headed. Temperatures up to 33 or 37°C (92 or 98°F) are suitable for range-of-motion and stretching exercise but not for serious swimming.
- Don't go swimming with a temperature, an open wound or if you have a history of uncontrolled seizures, or have either high or low blood pressure.

Heat

Heat reduces pain, and soothes and relaxes mind and body. It works by causing the blood vessels to expand (vasodilatation), increasing the blood flow to the area and generally speeding up the metabolism.

Heat is especially useful as a prelude to exercise because joints perform better when warmed up. There are a number of different devices for delivering heat, most related to the domestic bath and hot-water bottle. There are whirlpool baths, infra-red heat lamps, hot packs and electric heating pads. Heat application can be used in conjunction with gentle range-of-motion exercises as part of your exercise warm-up.

What you use depends on your preference, but bear in mind it is important not to overdo heat. Some people have the mistaken idea that hotter is better. It's not. If the skin begins to blotch, the heat is too great, and no matter how relaxing it is you should never fall asleep while using heat treatment.

The use of cold is favoured by some physiotherapists, and although it does not have the relaxing, psychological benefits associated with heat, in the case of seriously inflamed, swollen joints the benefit of a cold application may be greater than that of heat.

Don't forget to warm down

Sports experts emphasize the importance of warming down or cooling down after vigorous exercise to help reduce cramps and soreness in tired muscles. It also makes you more flexible, and helps prevent injury. The idea is that you don't get cold, but just cool down gently. So, if you do exercise vigorously, allow a few minutes at the end of the session to warm down with lighter exercise and stretching. A therapeutic massage also helps, and is wonderfully relaxing.

9

Becoming a parent

What if you have Sjögren's and are planning to become pregnant? Or if you are already a parent and have just been diagnosed? It is very easy to be afraid of not coping when you are in pain or facing your very first pregnancy, but with information, support and planning you can find ways to be a happy and fulfilled Sjögren's parent.

The main point is to inform your doctor if you are planning to become pregnant. Most pregnancies are straightforward, but in a very few cases you might need extra tests for certain rare conditions, described more fully below. If possible, ask to be referred to an obstetrician who is knowledgeable about Sjögren's, and make sure you have any necessary tests and treatments to optimize your chances of having a healthy baby.

Miscarriage

It has to be remembered that miscarriage is common, and can happen very easily even in cases where a woman is totally healthy. According to the Miscarriage Association in the UK, more than one in five pregnancies ends in miscarriage – that's around a quarter of a million in the UK each year. Whatever the cause – and often it is impossible to determine – most women find it deeply distressing to lose a baby in this way. Lack of support and information can play a major part in this, so if you have suffered miscarriage it may be worth contacting a support organization such as the Miscarriage Association (see Useful Addresses).

Some women report recurrent miscarriages which they feel are linked to Sjögren's syndrome. While research on this is not extensive, a few women with Sjögren's may have antiphospholipid antibodies, sometimes called anticardiolipin antibodies, which can be associated with recurrent miscarriages, especially during the second trimester of pregnancy. They may cause clots to form in the placenta, interrupting the flow of blood to the foetus. Fortunately, you can be tested for these, and treatments are available, in the form of either aspirin, heparin or prednisolone. This condition is usually called the antiphospholipid syndrome and is most commonly associated with lupus.

Can the baby inherit Sjögren's?

There is no proven hereditary link, although it is possible that a genetic tendency to Sjögren's may be passed on. However, experts believe that a trigger is still needed to turn it into an active syndrome. Research into this aspect of Sjögren's is being conducted in the USA and in Europe, including the UK. So, this should not be something you spend time worrying about, though you may want to discuss it with your doctor if you do have concerns.

Pregnancy

In the vast majority of cases, pregnancy is straightforward. However, rarely, in pregnancies in women with Sjögren's syndrome who also have antibodies to Ro and La (see p. 16), the antibodies cross the placenta and affect the baby, resulting in a condition called neonatal lupus.

In the vast majority of cases this is not serious and does not need treatment, as it usually disappears within a few weeks. Neonatal lupus is not to be confused with lupus (systemic lupus erythematosus) and doesn't develop into it.

In its mild and most common form, neonatal lupus may take the form of a rash, on the face and head or scattered over the body. This tends to appear a few days or weeks after birth, particularly after sun exposure, and usually disappears after a few more weeks as the mother's antibodies are slowly metabolized by the baby. As the rash looks much like any other baby rash, it can be identified by doing a blood test.

Another effect of neonatal lupus is a low blood count, perhaps resulting in anaemia. Again, this is seldom serious and usually resolves without treatment in a few weeks. Liver disease is another effect which again usually clears up soon after birth.

Much more rarely, the baby's heart may be affected, resulting in a heart rhythm abnormality known as congenital heart block. This is a disorder in which the electrical signal that regulates the unborn baby's heartbeat is disrupted by abnormal antibodies. As a result, the heartbeat becomes very slow. Even in mothers with the Ro antibody, this complication occurs in fewer than one in 100 pregnancies.

A normal heartbeat starts in the upper heart (the atria or auricles) and travels smoothly through to the bottom of the heart (the ventricles). In heart block, the atrial beat (about 140 times per minute in a newborn) cannot get through to the ventricles because scar tissue blocks its path. The ventricles then have to beat on their own (about 60 times per minute in a newborn). As the ventricle beat determines the pulse, the baby has an abnormally slow pulse.

This can be detected on scans from about 12–15 weeks of pregnancy. If the unborn baby has heart block but appears to be doing well – which is usually the case – either nothing is done, or a special form of cortisone is given that will go through the placenta to the baby, which may help the heart beat normally again.

If it doesn't, or if the baby is not doing well and is big enough to deliver (30 weeks into pregnancy or later), delivery is often the best way of handling the problem. After birth, many babies with congenital heart block lead normal lives with no treatment, but some need pacemakers.

However, it must be emphasized that the overall outlook is good for babies born to mothers with Sjögren's.

A blood test during pregnancy can identify anti-Ro and anti-La antibodies, and women who test negative can rest assured they will not have a child with neonatal lupus. Those who test positive for only the anti-Ro antibody should be aware of the possibility of rash and blood test abnormalities in the child, but should not worry unduly. For pregnant woman with both anti-Ro and anti-La antibodies, regular scans between weeks 15 and 25 of pregnancy can check the baby's heartbeat (foetal echocardiography), and if an abnormality is detected, specialist treatment will be arranged as soon as possible for the best outcome.

Karen

After two miscarriages, I became and stayed pregnant. I was delighted, until during a routine scan during my 28th week the doctor was unable to find the baby's heartbeat. A scan and a foetal echocardiogram discovered that the baby had a heart block, though his heart had appeared and did still appear normal. I immediately had a blood test which showed I had Sjögren's syndrome – the first time I'd ever heard of it. The doctors explained that certain blood markers in my system were able to pass over into my baby's body and so affect his heart. I was taken into hospital until week 34, when I had a caesarean to deliver the baby – some of the most anxious and depressing weeks of my life. Luckily he was fine, and continues to be healthy and fit, with no need of a pacemaker or any other type of treatment.

After the birth and flare-ups

In some cases, Sjögren's may flare after a birth, so it's a good idea to plan for this just in case. Have a look at the action plan for flare-ups in Chapter 6.

Your after-birth follow-up plan should include:

- seeing your family doctor regularly, and making any appointments you need with specialists;
- resuming exercise – again, with the advice of your doctor;
- discussing with your doctor which medications, if any, you should take and if you can breastfeed your baby while taking them;
- knowing how much activity you can handle and how you can pace yourself so as to avoid exhaustion and stress.

Adjusting to motherhood

Patricia, mother of two
Those first few weeks after delivery were nothing like I'd imagined them to be. I thought I'd be able to get all the rest I needed because the baby would be so tiny, and that the Sjögren's would take care of itself. Lack of sleep was the worst factor – it made me feel fluey and achy all the time. With my first baby, it took nearly six months for me to begin to adjust to my new life.

The combination of Sjögren's, loss of sleep and the sheer impact of having a new person to care for can be exhausting. Don't expect too much of yourself and do give yourself time to adapt to becoming a mother. Remember, mothers without Sjögren's suffer exhaustion and depression, too, but you may need to take extra care (see Postnatal depression, p. 74).

Taking care of yourself

- *Rest as much as you can.* If possible, take a nap when your child does. If you need to rest while your baby is awake, ask family, friends or a hired person to care for her.

- *Get help during the first two weeks at the very least, longer if you can.* Another pair of hands is invaluable, for doing the washing up or just for holding baby while you shower. Get help from family and friends and make sure they understand your condition. Encourage any older children to get involved and help. Think about employing somebody – maybe just a local teenager – to help you with the physical tasks of childcare.
- *Leave the housework.* Yes, the house will need cleaning, and you'll wonder how such a small being can generate so much laundry, but it can be put off. A nap can be much more beneficial than sorting the whites from the coloureds.
- *Put yourself first.* Make looking after yourself a priority. Let others take the baby for an hour, and relax in a warm bath or shower; get some sleep; have a nutritious meal or snack; or just spend some quiet time alone to recharge your battery.
- *Keep in touch.* Try and make time for old friends, even if it's just a chat on the phone or an email, and try and make new ones. Internet-based motherhood support groups are good, but real faces are even better. Look for local mother and baby groups or try and keep up with people you may have met at antenatal classes.

Postnatal depression

No one is quite sure what causes postnatal depression – some blame hormones, others the psychological and social upheaval of becoming a mother. But, while having a new baby should represent one of the happiest times of your life, it's true that some women – an estimated 10–20 per cent – feel extra vulnerable, sad or anxious after a birth. The enormous responsibility of a new baby to care for, combined with the strain of having a chronic condition and the sheer tiredness that can be involved, may be implicated. Family factors are also important, including your relationship with your partner and the level of support you may have from others.

On the third or fourth day after the baby is born, it's common to experience the baby blues – feeling weepy, sad or irritable for no real reason. This often coincides with the arrival of your milk and you may also run a slight temperature. Symptoms usually pass in a day or two.

It is important to distinguish the baby blues from postnatal depression, symptoms of which include:

- feeling miserable, sad and tearful – life is not worth living and you have nothing to look forward to;
- feeling that you can't cope;
- feeling guilty and irritable, snapping at your partner or other children;
- being constantly exhausted, and often with disturbed sleep, including early morning waking;
- worrying about the baby and/or your own health;
- being unable to concentrate on anything or having a poor memory;
- feeling that your baby is a stranger and not really yours;
- having no interest in sex;
- finding it difficult to make decisions;
- having no appetite *or* comfort eating.

If this is you, get help. Go to your family doctor or talk to your health visitor. Postnatal depression is treatable, by medication, counselling or both, and the sooner treatment starts, the better for you and your baby.

Babycare

Aim to organize tasks so you expend the minimum amount of energy and effort. For example, you may find it difficult or painful to bend down and pick up the baby, or may have a fear of dropping her. With time, you will find the babycare methods that work best for you – and bear in mind this is true of all mothers, whether they have Sjögren's or not. It takes time to learn how to bathe, feed and dress a new baby – all part of the process of adapting to motherhood.

Bathing
Put the baby bath so it's level with you, i.e. on a worktop or in the sink, so you don't have to lean over, kneel or reach up to bathe your baby. If it is in or near the sink, you can use a short hose or shower attachment to fill it. A wash mitt may help you wash your baby if you have hand problems.

Wear an apron with large pockets to hold shampoo, soap and other items.

Sit on a high stool next to the sink while bathing the baby. If your baby just needs a wash, put her in a car seat or bouncing chair.

Feeding

Use a pillow on your lap to support and raise your baby and make feeding easier. A chair with arm rests will support your arms while holding him. You may find it easier to breastfeed lying on your side, rather than sitting upright and holding the baby.

If your feet are stiff and you find it hard to get out of bed for night feeds, do gentle range-of-motion exercises, especially to your ankles, before rising at night (see Chapter 8 on exercise). Keep a comfortable pair of slippers next to your bed. Ask your partner to bring the baby to you, or to give the baby night-time feeds. This is easier if you are bottle feeding but it is possible to express breast milk into a bottle for night-time feeds, too.

If you have hand problems, ask a family member to prepare baby bottles in advance, and keep the bottles in the refrigerator for the day.

Lifting and carrying

If you suffer joint pain and stiffness, lift and hold the baby with the arms rather than the hands so as to lessen the strain on wrists and fingers. You may find it more comfortable to hold the baby close to you with both arms rather than with one.

Use a lightweight pram or buggy that is easy to push and not too low, so that you don't have to bend low to put your baby into it. A cot with low sides will make for easier picking up and lying down. If you raise the cot by placing it on a solid wood dais or similar, ensure the legs are firmly supported or secured so the cot can't wobble or move.

Don't put anything – baby included! – on the floor. If you place the baby on a waist-level surface such as a bed, do ensure you are there to keep close watch in case of accidents. Your baby may learn to roll by three months and can take you by surprise!

Other tips

- Use a wheeled trolley or similar to help you move equipment around the house.
- A front-worn sling may be better than holding the baby all the

time – for you, it can be less uncomfortable, and gives better posture and less likelihood of accidents. For your baby, it means closer contact and probably much less crying!

- Use room intercoms so you can hear your baby when he is sleeping. This will save you from walking to the baby's room every five minutes to check that he is all right.
- Keep items you need during the day for the baby, such as nappies and changes of clothes, in the area of your home where you will be for most of the time, such as the kitchen.
- Babies grow quickly. Think ahead about baby-proofing your home, for example covering electric sockets and fitting cupboards with locks, so you don't exhaust yourself chasing after a crawling baby.
- Discuss any problems with your health visitor or doctor to see if they can help you find solutions.

10

Coping with your feelings

Living with a condition such as Sjögren's involves uncertainty, which in turn can mean stress. The condition can vary tremendously, sometimes from day to day, as Laura explains:

> Every day is different. One day I wake up feeling fine, the next I may be debilitated by poor sight, itchy skin and aching limbs. My Sjögren's is certainly a mover and shaker! It started with very itchy skin and then a red swollen eye. My optician sent me off for arthritis tests, and meanwhile I developed a lump beneath my parotid gland at the side of my face. It's gone on from there, and frankly by now I don't know what to expect next. I can live a normal life – just about – but I'm always on the lookout for the next symptom.

People react in different ways to being diagnosed with Sjögren's.

Grief

Mandy was happily married and had a career as a midwife, which she loved. As she used her hands in her work a great deal, she took no notice at first when the last three fingers of her left hand were constantly sore. In the end the registrar at work persuaded her to see her own family doctor, and after blood tests she was told she had rheumatoid arthritis. She was then referred to a rheumatologist for further treatment. Her condition worsened as the pain moved into both hands, wrists, elbows, knees and ankles, and she began to feel extremely tired, more so than the usual fatigue after shift work. She was always run down, and caught every cold and flu that went around. She took long-term sick leave and was planning to give up her career. On the advice of another doctor at the hospital where she worked, she saw a different rheumatologist, who immediately diagnosed Sjögren's. For Mandy, the diagnosis meant grief as it threatened her job and meant the end of a certain personality she felt she had – happy and coping. In the end she took sick leave for nine months and then resumed on a part-time basis, which gave her a better balance of work and leisure.

Relief

Kimberley

I was so relieved to get a diagnosis because I can finally put a name to a never-ending series of health problems over the past five years. It is so good to know that it's not just all in my head and I'm *not* a hypochondriac.

Anger

Laura

I literally cry with anger. I feel that my illness contributed to the break-up of my most recent relationship and, frankly, I sometimes despair of ever being able to have a long-term sexual relationship. I feel as if I'm 100 years old and I'm only 23. I feel this illness is cheating me out of my life.

Delayed reaction

Christine

For a few years I dealt really well with the fact that I had a chronic condition, and managed to lead a relatively normal life by working round my symptoms – I was so used to them and I suppose I assumed they'd never worsen. Then life threw a few situations at me. First we relocated offices, which vastly added to my daily travelling, and then I was made redundant and didn't work for nearly a year. Then I had a miscarriage. Finally my father died unexpectedly. He was only 57. I think the combined stress of these life events influenced me. I certainly spiralled downhill in a period of around two years. Today I am learning to pace myself and take life much easier – I now have a local, part-time job – but the exhaustion and aches and pains are much worse, I seem to have chronic sinus problems, and my face keeps swelling up when I get overtired. I can only hope things get better and that I get back on the relatively even keel I was on previously.

Restoring a sense of control starts with gaining an understanding of your illness. Reading this book is an excellent start! What you know about your condition can make a difference in how you approach each day. So, aim to be as well informed as possible – ask your family doctor or specialist for information, or contact a support group like the British Sjögren's Syndrome Association (BSSA, see Useful Addresses, p. 90).

Another useful information tool for you and your doctor is a medical diary. In it, keep track of your visits to the doctor – when and why. In addition, maintain a list of treatments and medications and any side-effects. You may also want to include copies of your test results, as well as a record of symptoms, their severity and possible triggers.

Emotional ups and downs

Living with a chronic illness can involve a roller-coaster of emotions. There are several ways you can help even out the ups and downs:

- *Keep in touch* – don't shut yourself away from the world, and do make the most of family and friends. Don't keep your feelings to yourself. A friend can help you break through negative feelings and suggest alternative ways of thinking, feeling and behaving. Try and be with people even if you don't feel like talking. In particular, doing something for someone else boosts your self-esteem, helps you feel like a real person again, and offers relief from worries about what may happen to you.
- *Keep up ordinary everyday activities* – whether it's going to concerts, singing in the church choir or just meeting friends for lunch. Doing things you are used to or things you are good at establishes continuity that counteracts those feelings of disruption and loss.
- *Give yourself rewards* – make a list of things you enjoy, such as favourite videos, pieces of music, favourite foods, places in the country, the seaside or pets.
- *Find out as much as you can about your condition* – about Sjögren's syndrome in general, and your own state of health in particular. Try and learn your physical limits and the effects of the illness, as well as how to deal with any treatments. Try and ensure you have good communication with your doctors.
- *Talk to someone* – most of the unpleasant emotions that plague people with a chronic illness are better out than in. By acknowledging and talking about feelings you gain more insight into them, and are more able to change them for the better. You probably already have family, friends or colleagues with whom

you discuss your life, but additionally it can be helpful to look for people who also suffer from Sjögren's (see Useful Addresses for support organizations and internet links).

Dealing with depression

Depression is one of the most common complications of an ongoing or chronic illness such as Sjögren's. This is natural. Not only are there the physical effects, there is a psychological reaction to the illness. There may be loss of mobility and independence to contend with, and having a diagnosis of Sjögren's can change the way you see yourself and how you relate to others. In fact, it may require an in-depth re-evaluation of your whole self-image.

It's worth bearing in mind that depression can often make pain and fatigue worse, so aggravating the symptoms of Sjögren's; it can also increase any social isolation.

It is, however, quite possible to overlook the symptoms of depression, assuming that feeling depressed is normal for someone struggling with a serious, chronic illness. Symptoms of depression include:

- feeling sad or depressed, with loss of interest or pleasure in daily activities;
- significant weight loss or weight gain;
- sleep disturbances – sleeping too much or not being able to sleep;
- problems with concentration;
- apathy;
- feelings of worthlessness or guilt;
- fatigue or loss of energy;
- recurrent thoughts of death or suicide.

Just as with Sjögren's itself, early diagnosis and treatment for depression are essential. People who get treatment for depression that occurs at the same time as a chronic disease often experience an improvement in their overall medical condition and a better quality of life, and are more easily able to stick to their treatment plans.

Many antidepressant medicines are available to treat depression and can start to work within a few weeks, and more than 80 per cent of people with depression can be treated successfully with medicine, psychotherapy or a combination of both. These drugs work by altering the level of certain chemicals in the brain, which are responsible for transferring messages between brain cells.

Psychotherapy refers to a variety of techniques used to treat depression. It involves talking to a licensed professional who helps the depressed person understand his or her depression better, and regain a sense of control and pleasure in life.

One of the advantages of talking to professionals – not necessarily doctors, but those experienced in assessing psychological problems – is that they are able to judge whether your depression or anxiety is serious enough to be treated with drugs. Your GP can refer you to a counsellor, or you can contact a support organization (see Useful Addresses).

Dealing with anger and resentment

Not everyone with a diagnosis of Sjögren's will feel angry, but some people do. Perhaps you may be feeling, 'Why me? What did I do to deserve this? Why is life so unfair?' Again, this is a natural reaction and it is most helpful to acknowledge it.

It is quite natural to look for something to blame when bad things happen to you. Some people may 'take it out' on their doctors, because they seem slow and uncaring; others may blame employers or work colleagues for not understanding their problems; yet others may get annoyed with their family for not helping enough with domestic tasks – or because they start to treat you like an invalid and that makes you feel like one.

- Try and get the anger out, either to a close friend or to a therapist. Write it down – emailing others in an online support group is one tactic many people today have found helpful. (See Useful Addresses.)
- Try and channel some of your anger – anger is energy, so use it to try and solve the situations that are making you so cross. For example, you may need to discuss work issues with an employer or colleagues in a more assertive way, or you may need to be more assertive with your family and to set limits with them if necessary.

- Scale down your expectations. You are now someone coping with a chronic disease. That leaves less room for other things, or means other things take longer. One way to create more realistic expectations is to scale jobs down into small tasks – not 'I must clean the house' but 'Today I will clean the bathroom.' Only do the longer distance when the shorter becomes easy. And if and when you manage to build upon what you undertake, don't forget to congratulate yourself!

Managing feelings with your partner and family

It is natural to feel anger, sadness and frustration, and your partner or other family members may also go through the same emotions. A chronic illness affects not only you, but also the entire family. There are particular problems to be faced in dealing with people who depend on you: children, partners and parents. How do you rearrange your role from being someone who supports everyone else to being someone who needs support?

The first thing to do is to dismiss guilt. Tell yourself firmly that you have nothing to feel guilty about. No one is to blame for you getting Sjögren's – least of all you. The situation has to be dealt with, by you and by everyone involved with you. People who value you will not mind making adjustments.

If you are the sort of person whom others rely on, much of your self-esteem may depend on the role. Sjögren's requires that you give up some of this. But just as it may have given you satisfaction to be needed, by asking others to support you, you are giving them importance and a chance to be responsible and caring towards you. It can be an act of generosity to allow others to give to you.

Both you and your partner may find it helpful to consider the following suggestions:

- Accept your feelings. Don't berate yourself if you are sad or resentful. These feelings are normal as you adjust to the changes that follow the diagnosis of a chronic illness.
- Communicate your feelings with your partner. Share your fears and frustrations in an honest but caring way.
- Include your family in the process of dealing with the diagnosis and its aftermath. Share with any children in an age-appropriate

way – this can be just a few words of explanation for a smaller child, which can be enlarged upon as the children grow older. Whatever their age, they will cope much better if they have some understanding of what is going on. Give them the chance to share their own fears and resentments, too – sometimes children may blame themselves for what has happened, and it is important for them to air these and similar feelings.

- Explain to children if there will be any changes in their routine – for example, if you need to make arrangements for someone else to collect them from school sometimes.
- It can be very helpful for partners to establish a separate support network outside the immediate family, so they have a way of sharing private feelings about their other half's chronic illness.
- Get professional help if necessary. When adjusting to chronic illness, it may be helpful to seek the guidance of a professional counsellor to help each member of the family cope with the necessary changes in their own way.
- Get involved in the treatment process. As much as possible, be a partner to the patient. Go along on visits to the doctor. Learn as much as possible about the disease, its limitations, available treatments and helpful strategies to make life easier and more comfortable.
- Use a teamwork approach. Problem-solve together as you try to create a realistic plan for how to handle the children, housework, scheduling and social calendar. As partners, recognize the limitations of the illness and set realistic expectations and goals – what must be done, what should be done, what might be done. Don't forget to plan for fun times that allow you to stay close and connected.

How to help

Living with someone who has Sjögren's can be frightening and depressing, but there is much that partners, family and friends can do to help. (As stated at the front of this book, most people with Sjögren's are women, so we are referring to 'she' here.)

- Do your best to be supportive, give encouragement and offer hope. Be patient and understanding. Your help at this time is absolutely invaluable. Most importantly for you, be prepared to seek help, both for her and for yourself if you feel you need it.

- Ask her what she needs and how best you can help. It may be that she has a clear idea of what help is needed – perhaps you taking over the shopping for the week, or taking the children to school, acting as a mediator between her and her doctor, or just sitting and listening while she talks.
- Encourage her to accept help from others and to seek it if need be from the health visitor or GP. Offer to accompany her if you think it may help.
- Suggest she joins a support group such as the British Sjögren's Syndrome Association (BSSA, see Useful Addresses). Exchanging experiences with people in a similar position and realizing that you really are not the only one suffering can be an enormous relief. Again, this may not be something she may feel she wants to do at first, but as she begins to feel better she may change her mind. If it is appropriate you could offer to go with her.
- Offer help with practical arrangements such as childcare, cleaning, washing, ironing and so on.
- Be patient. Please remember that Sjögren's is an illness. She cannot help suffering the symptoms that she does. Hopefully she is doing all she can for herself to try and make herself think positively and feel better.
- Let her express her true feelings, even if it is not easy for you to hear what she has to say. You may feel that you are hearing the same things again and again, and wonder if it is really helping her. Some people need to talk about something endlessly; some people may not want to talk about it very much at all. Whatever suits that person is to be encouraged.
- Find out as much as you can about Sjögren's syndrome, especially if she is perhaps frightened of what she may find out if she explores, or just feels too ill to do so.
- Give her treats – a cuddle, a cup of tea in bed, a special phone call or text message.
- Ensure that she gets enough food and rest. You could try and leave a prepared meal for her in the fridge the evening before.
- Encourage her to be active – perhaps take a short walk together.
- Give her a massage. Don't worry, you don't need to be an expert, most of us aren't. Try some gentle stroking of her neck, shoulders and back to start with, or if you and she prefer you could massage her feet.
- Get help if you need it at any time – don't keep your problems to

yourselves. Talk to your doctor, or there are a number of organizations that are able to offer you advice and support, such as Carers UK and the British Sjögren's Syndrome Association (BSSA, see Useful Addresses).

- Last but not least, try not to slip into the age-old temptation of telling her to 'pull yourself together'. She will not appreciate it. If she could, she would – even though she may be applying the same advice to herself! Instead, reassure her of your love and support.

Positive thinking

There is some confusion about positive thinking and illness – a kind of uneasy feeling that if you think positive thoughts hard enough, you ought to be able to 'magic' your Sjögren's away, and that if it persists, it is your fault because you were not positive enough. Some people may fear that feeling sad or having negative feelings may delay their recovery or make the Sjögren's worse.

You may also be told by other people to 'think positive' if you feel low or tearful, or want to talk about the hard fact that you have a chronic illness for which there is no known cure. Such remarks from others can add to the confusion.

Being positive does not mean curing or banishing your Sjögren's, and it is not your fault if your illness persists! Being positive also does not mean you have to feel happy and cheerful all of the time – it is actually positive to acknowledge when you feel sad, tired or angry. You are allowed to state when you are finding life difficult, or just to have a good cry when it all gets too much. Tears are a natural response to distress and can be a healthy release for you.

Positive thinking means different things to different people, but generally it is about facing up to the Sjögren's. People do this in different ways. Some take a more active part in their treatment, reading all they can, surfing the internet, talking to lots of people. Others prefer to leave matters more in the hands of their doctors. Still others prefer to ignore the whole thing and just carry on as normally as possible.

Bear in mind that it is easier to feel positive if you are eating and sleeping well, and getting enough rest and exercise. You may also find it helpful to deal with any underlying psychological or emotional issues that may be gnawing away at your sense of wellbeing.

This said, when you focus your attention on positive thoughts, ideas and images, you do tend to feel better. The link between a positive attitude and good health is well documented. One study of psychosomatic medicine found that people with a positive attitude were less likely to catch colds than those who were depressed, nervous or angry. The study also found that uptight or sad people are more likely to complain of cold symptoms, even when they don't have a cold.

How to be more positive

- *Make a list of ten things you have accomplished on a daily basis –* small things, such as choosing a nice outfit for the day, tidying a room or ringing a friend.
- *Choose an 'accomplishment symbol' –* something you normally do each day that you endow with the power to represent an accomplishment. Your accomplishment symbol may be brushing your teeth, washing your face, shaving, having breakfast. Remember, it is something you are already doing, *not* something you think you should be doing. Whenever you do this each day, you can start to enjoy that sense of accomplishment.
- *Interpret events differently –* find the positive interpretation to the negatives in your life. If a negative thought comes to you, turn it round so the focus shifts from what you have lost to what you still have.
- *Exercise –* it's well known that exercise gives you a natural high by releasing natural body chemicals – endorphins – which appear to reduce pain and lift the spirits. Exercise also concentrates the mind because it involves effort and gives you less opportunity to indulge in unpleasant thoughts.

Conclusion: the future

Sjögren's syndrome is the second most common form of auto-immune disease after rheumatoid arthritis. Why do these bewildering diseases occur and what can be done to reverse or halt them? Research has a long way to go before finding answers. The root causes of immune diseases are likely to be combinations of factors, both genetic and environmental. About 75 per cent of auto-immune diseases are found in women, and women are more likely to get one immune disease if a family member has suffered too – for example, your mother may have had lupus, while you have Sjögren's. A genetic predisposition to such diseases seems evident, but it is not that strong – the vast majority of people who have a relative with an auto-immune disorder will remain free of disease.

Other factors need to be taken into account in research. Some auto-immune diseases are known to begin or worsen with certain triggers, such as viral infections or medication. The severity or pattern of an auto-immune disease may be influenced by the genes a person inherits. It is thought that hormones play a role in inducing auto-immune diseases; some cases suddenly improve during pregnancy, some flare-ups occur after delivery, while others will get worse during pregnancy, or flare up after menopause. Other less understood influences affecting the immune system and the course of auto-immune diseases include ageing and stress. All of these offer areas for future research in order to increase our understanding of auto-immune disease.

Research into Sjögren's is being pursued in many ways. Some workers are trying to unravel the genetic factors, while others are studying potential environmental triggers. Treatment research has focused on three main areas: first, to improve the efficacy and tolerability of artificial lubricants; second, to promote the secretion of the body's own tears and saliva; and third, to dampen down the body's immune and inflammatory responses.

Medical advances sometimes come from surprising sources – one of the most commonly used treatments for osteoporosis came from research into washing powders! – so who knows where the next breakthrough will come from?

But while scientific studies are ongoing, the most important researcher right now is you. By taking an active role in your treatment, noting your specific symptoms and finding out how best to deal with them, and exploring therapies and lifestyles that may help, you are well on the way to empowerment. And empowerment lies at the heart of healing.

Useful Addresses

UK

Sjögren's syndrome
British Sjögren's Syndrome Association (BSSA)
PO Box 10867
Birmingham
B16 0ZW
Helpline: 0121 455 6549
Tel: 0121 455 6532
Fax: 0121 455 6532 (please telephone before sending fax)
Email: kate@bssa.uk.net
Website: www.bssa.uk.net/regional.htm

Arthritis
Arthritis Care
18 Stephenson Way
London
NW1 2HD
Freephone helpline: 0808 800 4050
Tel: 020 7360 6500
Email: helplines@arthritiscare.org.uk
Website: www.arthritiscare.org.uk

National Rheumatoid Arthritis Society
Briarwood House
11 College Avenue
Maidenhead
Berkshire
SL6 6AR
Tel: 01628 670606
Email: enquiries@rheumatoid.org.uk
Website: www.rheumatoid.org.uk

Help for patients and carers

British Association for Counselling and Psychotherapy (BACP)
35–37 Albert Street
Rugby
CV21 2SG
For a list of BACP-accredited counsellors in your area, call 0870
443 5252
Email: bacp@bacp.co.uk
Website: www.bacp.co.uk

Carers UK
20–25 Glasshouse Yard
London
EC1A 4JT
Tel: 020 7490 8816
Fax: 020 7490 8818
Email: info@carersuk.org
Website: www.carersuk.org

Depression Alliance
35 Westminster Bridge Road
London
SE1 7JB
Tel: 0845 123 23 20 (calls charged at local rates)
Email for local groups: groups@depressionalliance.org
Website: www.depressionalliance.org

The College of Health
St Margaret's House
21 Old Ford Road
London
W2 9PL
Tel: 020 8983 1225
Website: www.collegeofhealth.org.uk
(Represents the interests of NHS patients in the UK)

The Miscarriage Association
c/o Clayton Hospital
Wakefield
West Yorkshire
WF1 3JS
Helpline: 01924 200799
Fax: 01924 298834
Email: info@miscarriageassociation.org.uk
Website: www.miscarriageassociation.org.uk

North America

Canada

Sjögren's Syndrome Association Inc.
(Association du Syndrome de Sjögren Inc.)
Tel: (514)934-3666, (877)934-3666

USA

American College of Rheumatology
1800 Century Place, Suite 250
Atlanta
GA 30345
Tel: 404-633-3777
Fax: 404-633-1870
Email: acr@rheumatology.org
Website: www.rheumatology.org

The National Institute of Arthritis and Musculoskeletal and Skin
Diseases (NIAMS)
Information from:
NIAMS/National Institutes of Health
1 AMS Circles
Bethesda
MD 20892-3675
Website: www.nih.gov/niams/

National Institutes of Health
Sjögren's Syndrome Clinic
10 Center Drive, MSC 1190
Building 10, Room 1N113
Bethesda
MD 20892-1190
Tel: 301-435-8528
Website: www.ninds.nih.gov

Sjögren's Syndrome Foundation
8120 Woodmont Avenue, Suite 530
Bethesda
MD 20814-1437
Tel: 301-718-0300
Fax: 301-718-0322
Email: ssf@sjogrens.org
Website: www.sjogrens.org

Web addresses

Tips on internet searching

While the internet is a source of useful information, you do need to be discriminating and to read some pages with reservations. Some useful tips: the boxes at the side of the page are paid for, so may have a specific focus or even a product to push. The suffix .org implies a charity or an organization whose primary focus is not commercial. The suffix .ac or .edu implies an academic or educational site, likely to be well informed but possibly narrow or esoteric in focus. Perhaps the most useful function of the internet is its ability to put you in touch with others who live with Sjögren's.

Almark's page
http://www.almark.net/sjogrens_syndrome_home.htm

American Autoimmune Related Diseases Association
Website: www.aarda.org

The British Pain Society
Website: www.britishpainsociety.org

The Fibromyalgia Association, UK
Website: www.fibromyalgia-associationuk.org
Information on fibromyalgia.

http://lynne-sjogrens.org
Personal web page where several people share their experiences of Sjögren's.

http://www.myalgia.com/sjogrens.htm
Information on fibromyalgia and Sjögren's.

Further Reading

Carsons, Stephen and Harris, Elaine K., *The New Sjögren's Syndrome Handbook*, Oxford University Press, Oxford, 1998.

Dauphin, Sue, *Understanding Sjögren's Syndrome*, Pixel Press, 1993.

Rumpf, Dr Teri and Hammit, Kathy, *The Sjögren's Syndrome Survival Guide*, New Harbinger Publications, Oakland, California, USA, 2003.

The Official Patient's Sourcebook on Sjögren's Syndrome: A Revised and Updated Directory for the Internet Age, Icon Health Publications, 2002 (for internet users).

Sjögren's Syndrome: Advisory Guide for Patients and Doctors, order from the British Sjögren's Syndrome Association (BSSA; see Useful Addresses).

Index